Modified Inferior Turbinoplasty

Paolo Gottarelli

Modified Inferior Turbinoplasty

A New Surgical Approach

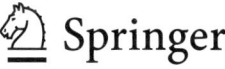 Springer

Paolo Gottarelli
Rhinoplasty Surgeon
Bologna, Italy

This is the English version of the Italian edition published under the title *La turbinoplastica inferiore modificata*, by Paolo Gottarelli
© Springer-Verlag Italia 2012

The Publisher gratefully acknowledges the support of Ars Medica Italia for the images

ISBN 978-88-470-2441-0   e-ISBN 978-88-470-2442-7

DOI 10.1007/978-88-470-2442-7

Springer Milan Heidelberg New York Dordrecht London

Library of Congress Control Number: 2011940270

© Springer-Verlag Italia 2012

9 8 7 6 5 4 3 2 1   2012   2013   2014

Cover design: Ikona S.r.l., Milan, Italy
Typesetting: Ikona S.r.l., Milan, Italy
Printing and binding: Grafiche Porpora S.r.l., Segrate, Milan, Italy

Printed in Italy

Springer-Verlag Italia S.r.l. – Via Decembrio 28 – I-20137 Milan
Springer is part of Springer Science+Business Media

Preface

Since the beginning of my medicine studies I have always been fascinated by the possibility of changing facial features and, with this concern, rhinoplasty has always attracted me, until it has become the main goal of my professional career. After my military service as an Alpine Troops officer at the Italian frontier, at the age of 27 I became physician assistant at the Plastic Surgery Department ruled by Dr Carlo Cavina, who initiated me into practice of nose surgery through the first essential surgical concepts. Nine years later, as plastic surgery head physician assistant, I started to go and visit the most important nasal surgeons in the world, trying to widen the concepts and the techniques learned initially.

I still remember Fernando Ortiz Monasterio (1923) who, after a tennis match, explained to me the advantages of percutaneous greenstick osteotomy. It was May 19, 1986, and since that date I have only been using that method to draw the nasal bones nearer after nasal hump reduction or simply to correct a post-traumatic asymmetry – and always using a 2 mm straight osteotome.

I remember fundamental meetings with Ralph Millard (1919) and his 33 principles that even nowadays I consider an indispensable guide for any (not necessarily plastic) surgeon. In 1988 I was impressed by the technically over-careful rhinoplasty intervention performed by John B. Tebbetts in Dallas, Texas. Ruled by a strict logic, this young surgeon was able to stand up to the most famous nasal surgeons such as Jack Sheen. This convincing logic led him to write, in 1988, a beautiful book about the reasons why primary rhinoplasty should always be dealt with using open approach, with the help of a very sophisticated method. And it was in Dallas, Texas, that a group of excellent surgeons was created, led by Jack Gunter and followed by Steve H. Byrd, Rod J. Röhrich, John B. Tebbetts, and many others. With their lectures and guidelines collected in two volumes entitled *Dallas Rhinoplasty*, they transformed the open approach into the best method to treat every part of the nose, not only in secondary cases, but even more in primary rhinoplasty cases: thanks to improved performance accuracy, primary cases did not evolve to secondary cases prompted by frequent relapse.

Back 1989, I started presenting the results obtained with Tebbetts's technique at the major conferences. In April 1994 I won the first prize at the *Congresso Italiano di videochirurgia plastica* (Italian Congress of Videoplastic Surgery), three months before Tebbetts published his work about Force Vector Tip Rhinoplasty (FVTR) (Shaping and positioning the nasal tip without structural disruption, a new, systematic approach. Plast Reconstr Surg 94:61–77). The awarded video at that congress presented, with a two year follow-up, the solution to a serious problem of idiopathic unilateral valve insufficiency, only using Tebbetts' technique with cartilage grafts and peculiar stitches.

In 1997, with Tebbetts's authorization, I organized and led in Bologna the first multimedia live videolecture on nasal surgery, using this method. In the same year I had the idea to treat turbinate hypertrophy as a plastic surgeon would do with breast hypertrophy, by harmoniously reducing all three anatomic compartments of the turbinate itself, and then rebuilding it with accurate sutures so as to avoid the development of cicatricial synechiae, bleeding and, most of all, without the use of swabs. This method proved to be fundamental for patient well-being, because it provided a faster and, above all, definite recovery.

Since then I performed modified inferior turbinoplasty (MIT) on patients with functional diseases and when aesthetic surgery was required. All this with the aim to re-balance the loss of space inside the choanae caused by reduction rhinoplastic surgery that unavoidably affects their function.

Later, in 2003, I introduced the MIT technique at the Teknon Clinic in Barcelona, to an authoritative group of nasal surgeons headed by Eugene M. Tardy, Jr., who used and wrote words of admiration for this technique, that was actually derived from one of his teachers, Dr. Howard P. House.

One year later, in 2004, I was invited by Jaime Planas to hold three lectures and a live surgery at the homonymous clinic in Barcelona during the two-year course organized there. I remember the exact words that Planas told me: "Dear Gottarelli, I know many surgeons who do beautiful noses, but very few also know how to make them breathe. If it is true that your technique works, you've brought up a sore point, and this is why I've invited you to our course".

In the following years, I made the new concept of nasal surgery more and more real, and defined it the "Global Rhinoplasty". Global Rhinoplasty is based not only on MIT, but also on the so-called "Structural Rhinoplasty" introduced by Dean Toriumi and on the above-mentioned FVTR by John B. Tebbets.

This is what the most modern and up-to-date methodology can offer in this field, overcoming not only the controversies between open and closed rhinoplasty, but also the distinction between pure functional surgery and pure cosmetic surgery. In these interventions, elements belonging to either approach may be recognized. For this reason, considering the dichotomy between functional and cosmetic surgery as outdated, it is more correct to speak about *nasal job* or Global Rhinoplasty. This innovative approach of thinking and performing nasal surgery has not failed to meet the approval by hundreds of patients, who this year established a nonprofit association (*Io Respiro* Onlus, meaning "I Breathe"), committed to spread, among other goals, information on this new method. Moreover, a new training school for nose surgery has been created too; its goal is to train a new generation of nasal surgeons with experience in plastic surgery, otolaryngology, maxillo-facial surgery, endoscopic surgery and microsurgery.

Paolo Gottarelli

With sincere gratitude I would like to dedicate this book to those who followed me along my professional and medical career, namely: all my colleagues, the operating room personnel, as well as my staff who supported me with enthusiasm. In particular, I have to thank the gift of life and the strength my parents gave me, to whom I will eternally be grateful.

Contents

Introduction

What is described in this volume about the new method for hypertrophic inferior turbinate treatment is nothing but the logic consequence of a series of innovations that come from very far. One by one, these innovations have allowed for treatment of the nose in all of its parts and functions with greater precision and result predictability. In order to get through this journey easily, it is necessary, as usual, to follow the historical steps of this slow but inexorable evolution.

None of the expert surgeons who wish to give a real meaning to their work can ignore this. In 1921, Aurel Rethi (1884-1976) paved the way with his columellar incision. However, this first "open" rhinoplasty followed the same stages as traditional rhinoplasty, suggested by Jacques Joseph (1865-1934). This meant that the actual benefits that the open approach allowed for could not be appreciated, with an additional scar on the columella that made, at that point, the real advantages fruitless.

This argumentation, opposed to the open approach, has been supported for many years by those who did not want to consider what happened from Rethi's method onwards, a revolutionary event, from all viewpoints. Following this sterile and obstinate controversy, many opposers prevented two generations of surgeons from taking a new road so full of satisfaction and success.

It is thanks to Ante Sercer (1896-1968), a Croatian professor, that the new technique with the open approach, which he called "decortication", was filled with anatomical and functional meanings for the first time. Actually, this naming was not very suitable, because it contributed to raising fears and suspicion in surgeons. In fact, the term "decortication" sounds a bit frightful and reminds us of the treatment for rhinophyma, that is the complete ablation of the thickened skin layers of the nose.

Besides this unfortunate definition, a second issue that prevented the diffusion of this method was the simultaneous work by another great teacher and surgeon, Maurice H. Cottle (1898-1981), who was much more diplomatically able to become popular with his appreciated method. Sercer's activity was so prolific that his most promising student, Ivo Padovan (1922-2010), was responsible for the continuation of this procedure, spreading this method overseas, in the USA. However, for twenty years, the diffidence among most American surgeons prevailed, with the exception of Jack R. Anderson (1917-1992) and Wilfred S. Goodman, who not only began to appreciate this new technique, but also presented their cases in several medical conferences. Anderson subsequently published the first article on this new approach and defined this method "Open Rhinoplasty": this new terminology, instead of Sercer's "decortication", was not frightening, and raised the curiosity of nasal surgeons.

From 1980 onwards, an increasing number of surgeons became active in this new field and, since the mid-nineties, "Open Rhinoplasty" was taught in all schools of specialization in Nasal Surgery overseas.

A new generation of surgeons was being formed, and thanks to them the possible interventions on aesthetic and functional diseases widened enormously. Today an overwhelming majority of surgeons experience the Open Approach with their patients' total approval and satisfaction.

From 1997 till now the number of patients operated on using this approach has reached 5,000.

The History of Rhinoplasty

The history of nasal surgery dates back to the mists of time. In the so-called "Edwin Smith ancient Egypt papyrus", purchased by the American antiquarian Edwin Smith (1822-1906) in Luxor in 1862, there are descriptions of the diagnosis and treatment of nasal deformities dating back to about 3,000 years ago.

In 800 BC the Indian physician Sushruta described in his Ayurvedic medicine book *Sushruta Samhita* surgical interventions conducted on more than 300 patients performed on the banks of the Ganges, as well a technique for nasal reconstruction. In the sixteenth century, the Bolognese physician Gaspare Tagliacozzi (1545-1599) used surgical reconstruction techniques to correct disfigured noses. In the following centuries, the science and art of rhinoplasty remained substantially stagnant until the nineteenth century, when the first plastic surgery pioneers appeared, such as doctor Johann Friedrich Dieffenbach (1792-1847) from Berlin who, in 1840, used a skin flap to cover the nasal back.

The first report of a modern endonasal rhinoplasty – published on Medical Record, 1887, June 4, *The Deformity Termed 'Pug Nose' and Its Correction by a Simple Operation* – was written by the American physician John Orlando Roe (1848-1915). In 1892 another American surgeon, Robert F. Weir (1838-1927), described step-by-step the rhinoplasty techniques for correction of misshapen noses.

In 1898, the orthopedic surgeon Jacques Joseph (1865-1934) presented his revolutionary concepts of nasal surgery at the Medical Society of Berlin. Many rhinoplasty surgery applicants traveled to Germany to learn his innovative techniques, to the point that he is considered the father of rhinoplasty. Many of the basic maneuvers of modern rhinoplasty are essentially the same as those described by Joseph two centuries ago.

Thanks to the work of surgeons such as Gustave Aufricht (1894-1980), Joseph Safian (1886-1983) and Samuel Fomon (1889-1971), these techniques

Paolo Gottarelli, *Modified Inferior Turbinoplasty* © Springer-Verlag Italia 2012

have further spread, in particular in the US. Fomon was the one who held the lectures and rhinoplasty courses that contributed to training many of the modern rhinoplasty surgeons, such as Maurice H. Cottle (1898-1981) from Chicago and Irving B. Goldman (1898-1975) from New York.

In the relatively short history of modern rhinoplasty, many experts have contributed to progress in this field through the development and refinement of new techniques. The continuing sharing and divulgation of rhinoplasty techniques have helped to improve the results on patient faces. Many patients who undergo nasal surgery are often only motivated by aesthetic reasons, but also frequently for concurrent respiratory disorders. And here comes the need for simple and multifaceted surgical techniques, where MIT will prove to have the utmost importance.

Well-Being and Respiration **2**

Today, well-being and fitness are well-known topics, but minor attention is still paid to two of the most vital functions of our health: feeding and breathing.

It is now recognized that a whole series of diseases having a highly social impact, cancer included, depends on lifestyle, food and atmospheric environmental conditions. The reason is due to the fact that our phenotype, the mutant and variable part of our DNA, represents the larger fraction of DNA and is strongly conditioned by our living habits. The most recent progress in cancer treatment comes exactly from the possibility of correcting DNA changes, by repairing the altered protein chains. The concept of reversibility is therefore predominating even in case of neoplastic diseases.

If we can live 40 days without eating and four days without drinking, we can survive four minutes at longest without breathing: this clearly accounts for the power and importance of respiration. Correct respiration slows down, filters, heats and humidifies the air breathed in through by the nose. Later on we will see the mechanisms through which all these important processes occur, but we must also underline the importance and the necessity of nasal respiration in order not to expose bronchi and pulmonary alveoli to a sudden and excessive air loading, as occurs any time one breathes through open mouth.

It is known that those who breathe through their mouth only, develop not only upper airway inflammatory diseases, but also severe bronchial, lung and even heart diseases more frequently. We know how many sleep disorders affect a huge amount of people, from ordinary roncopathy (snoring) to much more severe sleep apneas, and to the regular use (or even "abuse") of nasal vasoconstrictors that represent the only way to decongest the inferior hypertrophic turbinates for these patients, with the risk of developing consequent alterations of the nasal mucosa leading to the onset, in some cases, of hypertension. For these patients, MIT is able to solve the problem definitively.

Paolo Gottarelli, *Modified Inferior Turbinoplasty* © Springer-Verlag Italia 2012 5

Another important item regards child health; sometimes these patients are hurriedly defined as "allergic", instead of being visited by a specialist able to detect the presence of abnormalities or defects of the upper airways, like a septum deviation or an inferior turbinate hypertrophy. Hence, it should be stressed that even in these cases surgical intervention could be taken into consideration. Subjects should have to be selected in advance, with the utmost respect for their still-growing functional structures.

Moreover, we should not underestimate the occurrence of nasal and breathing symptoms in subjects who practice sports, both at amateur and professional level, which can limit their competitive performances by exposing them to frequent episodes of colds or inflammation of the respiratory tree (pharyngitis, bronchitis, etc.) and real sports performance handicaps such as the difficulty for divers in performing the Valsalva maneuver for compensation.

Poor blood oxygenation caused by alterations in the upper respiratory tract (particularly in the nose) is inevitably associated with social relationship disorders characterized by difficulties in concentration and performance, as well as sleep disorders followed by drowsiness during the day. But there are even negative effects on automatic mechanisms such as swallowing, conditioned by the presence of congenital or secondary nasal malformations, such as post-traumatic nasal septum deviations.

Nasal Anatomy and Function

3

3.1 Embryological Development

At the fourth week of gestational growth, the cells of the neural crest (where the nose will be formed) begin to migrate caudally towards the midface. Two symmetrical nasal placoderms (rudiments of the olfactory epithelium) develop; afterwards, they will be divided by the nasal pits into medial and lateral processes (rudiments of the superior lip and nose). The medial processes will form the septum, filter and nasal premaxilla; the lateral ones, instead, will form the lateral nose structure; finally, the stomodeum (the anterior ectodermal portion of the intestinal tract) will develop to form the mouth below the nasal structure. A nasobuccal membrane separates the mouth (lower oral cavity) from the nose (upper nasal cavity). When the olfactory pits deepen, the choanae develop, putting in communication the nasal cavity with the nasopharinx (Fig. 3.1).

At the tenth week, the cells differentiate into muscular, cartilaginous and bone tissue. Any change occurring during this early stage of facial embryogenesis will considerably affect the fetus with palatoschisis, cleft lip, choanal atresia, sinus aplasia, polyrhinia etc.

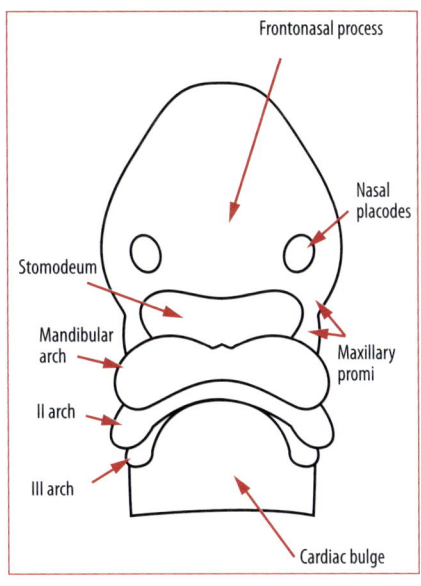

Fig. 3.1 Embryological development at the fourth week

3.2   Anatomical Structures

With the perspective of performing a corrective plastic surgery, the following anatomical components should be taken into consideration.

3.2.1   Soft Tissues of the Nose

Skin
The skin surface of the nose can be divided into three anatomic units:
- *upper third*: the skin of the upper portion of the nose, thin and relatively extendible (flexibility and mobility), closely adheres to the underlying osteocartilaginous structure;
- *middle third*: the skin of the nasal dorsum is the thinnest and least distensible, because it is closely adherent to the underlying anatomical structures;
- *lower third*: in addition to being particularly rich in sebaceous glands, the skin of the lower portion of the nose is similar to that of the upper third.

Mucosa
The vestibule is characterized by a mucous lining of squamous epithelium that, penetrating towards the inside, turns into transitional epithelium and then into cylindrical respiratory epithelium. It is a tissue rich in seromucous glands capable of maintaining upper airway humidification and protecting the airways from the pathogens in the atmosphere.

Muscles
Nose movements are controlled by four groups of facial and neck muscles deeply located beneath the subcutaneous layer and connected with the superficial muscolo-aponeurotic system (SMAS):
- the elevator muscle group;
- the depressor muscle group;
- the compressor muscle group;
- the dilator muscle group.

3.2.2   Aesthetic Nose Structure

Before planning, preparing and executing any nasal surgery, it is necessary to divide the external structure of the nose into subunits and aesthetic segments in order to help the plastic surgeon to determine exactly the size, extension and topographic location of defects or deformities to be corrected (Fig. 3.2):

- aesthetic nasal subunits:
  - lobule or tip of the nose
  - columella
  - right alar base
  - right alar wall
  - left alar wall
  - left alar base
  - dorsum of the nose
  - right dorsal wall
  - left dorsal wall
- aesthetic nasal segments:
  - dorsum of the nose
  - sidewalls
  - tip
  - soft triangle
  - ala nasi
  - columella.

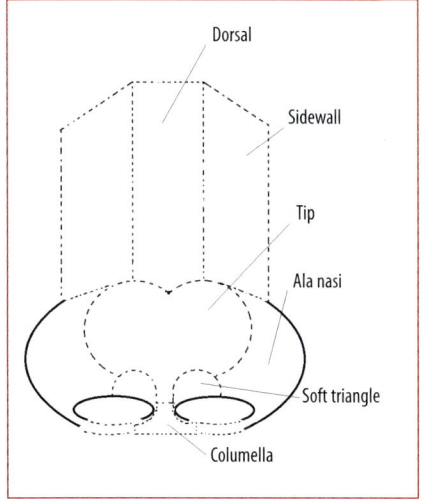

Fig. 3.2 External structure of the nose divided into aesthetic segments

3.2.3 Nose Bone Structure

In the antero-superior part of the splanchnocranium lies the **nasal bone**, formed by a thin, quadrilateral symmetric bone lamina. It varies in size and shape from individual to individual, closing the nasal cavities upwards and frontwards. Along with major, minor and accessory alar cartilages, it forms the external nose structure.

It is connected superiorly with the frontal bone, laterally with the maxilla and medially with its contralateral homologous through harmonic sutures. It is also connected with the ethmoid perpendicular lamina, and from their union, inferiorly and frontally on the median plane, the antero-superior nasal spine develops. The latter has two surfaces and four edges: the lower edge helps to define, at the upper level, the piriform orifice of the nose.

The **nasal septum** is a flat wall, pentagonal in shape, theoretically equidistant from the side wall in all its endonasal areas. It divides the inner nose into two compartments, forming the medial wall with an area of 30-35 cm^2.

The septum is made of a patchwork of structures (membrane, cartilage, bone) covered with cutaneous and mucous elements. Proceeding in the antero-posterior direction, the septum is composed by the columella (semi-rigid), membranous septum (flexible), septal cartilage (semi-flexible) and by the osteoseptum (rigid, albeit with some flexibility at the osteocartilaginous joints).

In addition to the basic components (cartilage, quadrangular, vomer, ethmoid perpendicular lamina), the columella, membranous septum, inferior nasal spine, premaxilla, maxillary nasal ridges, palatine bone nasal ridges, the sphenoid nasal ridge, frontal nasal ridge and medial processes of the nasal bones should also be considered as components of the septum. The core of this patchwork is represented by the premaxilla and its connections with the quadrangular cartilage and vomer.

The septum has four edges or angles: inferior, caudal, anterior or dorsal, and posterior. The anterior septal angle is located at the junction of the caudal and dorsal margins. The caudal edge has a curved profile and defines an angle – the inferior septal angle – at the junction between the middle and posterior thirds, that measures 45-55° approximately.

At the infero-caudal level, the septum rests on the inferior nasal spine (maxilla-premaxilla) behind which the premaxillary and alar ridges, maxillary and palatine ridges form the inferior bone septum. At the antero-superior level lies the quadrangular cartilage, contained within the septal cavity or area, lined with perichondrium. The cartilage of the septum is subdivided posteriorly into vomer and perpendicular lamina. This lamina should theorctically have a mid-sagittal direction, but it is often distorted by large-radius curvature. The superior portion of the perpendicular lamina is rarely pneumatized by the frontal septum. At the superior level, the frontal spine and the nasal bone processes form the cephalic septum, which completed the nasal dorsum.

The nasal septum represents the common element between cavities and nasal pyramid. Anatomically, it plays an essential role in the architecture of the external pyramid: the bone portion supports the nasal bones, while the cartilaginous septum represents the cartilaginous nasal dorsum. The osteocartilaginous components of the anterior septum significanty contribute to the architecture of the nasal valve area. An oblique deviation of the inferior nasal spine, premaxilla or anterior vomer can alter the shape of each nasal valve area. A reduction in the caudal edge height of the septal cartilage, at the level of the supporting area extending from the premaxilla to the dorsum, leads to a reduction in the *os internum* diameter, therefore causing a lowering of the septum-triangular junction.

The sidewalls of the nose contain three pairs of shell-shaped small bones: the **curled bones** (nasal conchae) or superior, medium and inferior **turbinates**. The inferior nasal turbinate defines, in the inner portion of the nasal choanae, the superior meatus (together with the medium nasal concha) and the inferior meatus, i.e. the area between the concha itself, the horizontal jaw portion (palatine process) and the horizontal palatal plate, extension of the process itself.

3.3   Functional Anatomy

The normal airway pattern is basically determined by the shape and size of the nasal cavities. Therefore, any difference in shape and size in the internal nose, both isolated or associated, causes an aerodynamic nasal discomfort, which is mainly characterized by obstructive disorders. The endonasal volume is a three-dimensional dynamic space constantly changing as it is influenced by environmental, hormonal, nervous and age-related factors. Therefore, the nose acts as a variable airflow resistor, whose resistance is made up of a constant and some variable components. The constant component is represented by the osteo-cartilaginous structure of the nasal cavities. The variable ones are vascular (degree of submucosal vascular plexus filling) and muscular (dilator muscle activity).

The volume can be divided into six parts:
- vestibular volume (or Cottle's area n. 1);
- valvular volume (or Cottle's area n. 2);
- attic (or Cottle's area n. 3);
- volume of the anterior turbinate (or Cottle's area n. 4);
- volume of the rear of the turbinates (or Cottle's area n. 5);
- choanal opening and nasopharynx.

The nasal septum represents the medial wall of endonasal volumes. These volumes can be modified through surgical procedures carried out for functional and/or aesthetic purposes. The major nasal resistive segments are located in the first 3.5 cm of nasal airway, as they are the vestibular and valvular segments of the nasal cavity. They are represented by the columella footplate, the rounded vestibule on the latero-caudal edge of the lateral crus, the superior *cul-de-sac*, the triangular cartilage-septum structure, the piriform opening floor and the head of the inferior turbinate.

3.4   Histology

From a histological viewpoint, the walls of the nasal cavities are made of 14 different kinds of tissue, each of them with a different healing capacity:
- cutaneous;
- subcutaneous;
- adipose tissue;
- connective tissue;
- nerves;
- arteries and veins;
- hyaline cartilage of the septum. Its biomechanical behavior depends on the properties and distribution of major components such as collagen

fibers, elastic fibers, chondrocytes, proteoglycan units, hyaluronic acid and water. These components have a complex interaction, which is the basis of a balanced system of forces (*internal interlocked stress system*), whose resultant is equal to zero: the outer layers maintain the inner layers under pressure and this condition provides the cartilage with its peculiar resilience;
- perichondrium;
- submucosa;
- bone;
- periosteum;
- respiratory mucosa (ciliated epithelium and related glands);
- mucocutaneous junction at the nostrils (subject to potential concentric stenosis-related contraction);
- chondro-osseous joint girdle of the septum.

The process of tissue healing depends on trauma dimension and severity. The tissues with fast recovery skills (skin, subcutaneous, connective, muscle and mucosa) heal forming a variable amount of cicatricial connective tissue, which exerts an unequal but constant traction twisting tissues with slow recovery skills (cartilage and bone).

3.5   Nasal Function

We have seen how important the nasal function is, which is reduced only because of an altered nasal anatomy. In particular, a correct nasal respiratory function depends on the morphology of at least three anatomical structures of the nose:
- nasal septum;
- nasal valve;
- inferior turbinates.

To these three anatomical structures we have to add a fourth one, which comes into play more infrequently and affects the health of the cavities in proximity and continuity to the nose:
- the paranasal sinuses.

When the mucosa lining these cavities gets sore, *sinusitis* (maxillary, frontal, etc.) arises; in order to avoid this disease, it is important that the septum cartilage (the most prominent) and the bone cartilage (posterior) are lined up as much as possible. Nasal septum deviations, besides causing a stenosis in one of the two nasal fossae (choanae), leads to the so-called *compensatory hypertrophy of the inferior turbinate* on the side opposite to the deviated fossa (Fig. 3.3).

The purpose of this compensation mechanism is to slow down the air

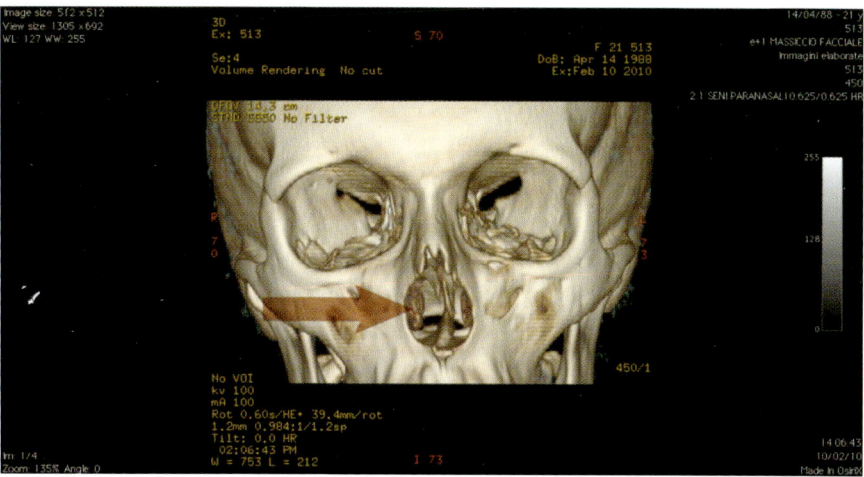

Fig. 3.3 Imaging of the facial skeleton and paranasal sinuses: compensatory hypertrophy of the bone

coming in too fast, which becomes too cold for this larger portion. As a result, quite paradoxically, the quality of breathing worsens, especially at night when the hypertrophic inferior turbinate is filled with more blood, thus occluding the choana concerned.

The *nasal valve* is, however, a delicate anatomical component that, in case of nasal plaster, is opened by lifting the skin at the level of the lateral or triangular cartilages of the nose that represent the middle part of the nose.

For surgical purposes, therefore, the nose can be briefly divided into three parts: the upper part, represented by the *nasal bones*, the intermediate part, with *lateral or triangular cartilages*, and the lower part, represented by *alar cartilages* that shape and support the tip of the nose.

The Inferior Turbinates

4

The nasal cavities are completely covered with mucus, firmly adherent to the periosteum and perichondrium of the underlying osteocartilaginous skeleton.

There are two distinguishable kinds of mucosa:

- the **respiratory mucosa**, pink and moist, that covers most of the surface. It is a pseudostratified columnar epithelium with cilia that move the airflow towards the rhinopharynx; mingled within are the caliciform muciparous glands, which produces the mucus that drapes the nasal mucosa for protective purposes; in the lamina there are glands with mixed serous-mucous secretion. Into the deeper layer, a cavernous tissue of the nasal mucosa is located, made of large, grossly dilated veins;

- the **olfactory mucosa**, smooth and yellowish, that covers the olfactory region, surrounded by the superior turbinate, superior meatus and part of the olfactory cleft, between the septum and the free edge of the middle turbinate. The epithelium of this mucosa is made of three different cells:
    - *Schultze's olfactory cells*, which are actual neurons with a proximal neuritic extension afferent to the first cranial nerve, and a distal dendritic extension, from where small branches on the mucosal surface depart;
    - *supporting cells*, cylindrical and very tall, each in close contact with the other;
    - *basal cells*, in contact with the basilemma; they can substitute the yellow-colored supporting cells.

In the *tunica propria* lie Bowman's olfactory glands, which produce serous secretions.

In this context we find the inferior turbinates, dynamic structures that are entitled to divert the nasal airflow and create a first resistance barrier in order to allow the supplying vascular system to "condition" the external airflow before entering the lungs (Fig. 4.1a,b).

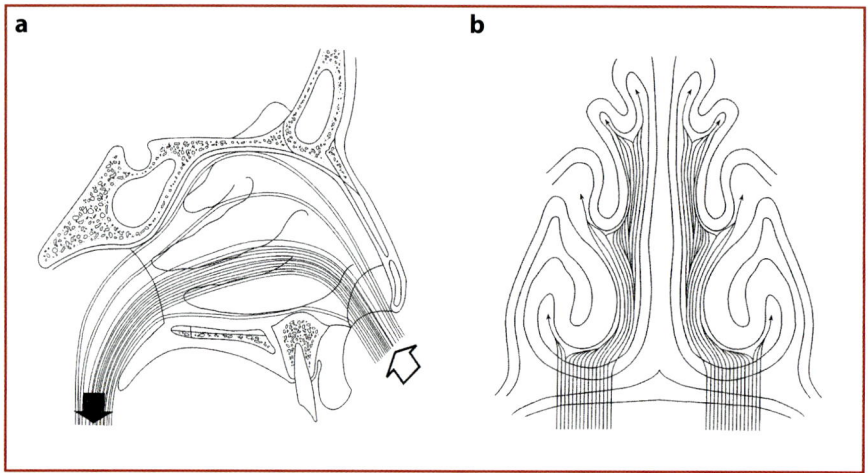

Fig. 4.1 Trajectory of inspiratory airflow inside the nasal conchae in sagittal (**a**) and frontal (**b**) projections

These structures are rather bulky (4-7 cm long, 2 cm large), located in the critical area of the nasal valve near the intermediate septum; they are made of trabecular bone, supplied by a thick net of capillaries and lined with mucocavernous tissue.

Examination of the nose by anterior rhinoscopy is capable of depicting the size, morphology and color of the inferior turbinates, as well as the pathophysiologic features of the nasal mucosa and the mucosal secretion. Administration of a vasoconstrictor (e.g., oxymetazoline hydrochloride) and an anaesthetic spray (tetracaine), may help to understand if the obstruction is caused by a simple mucosal congestion or, conversely, by anatomical changes such as an underlying trabecular hypertrophy.

All this considered, the indication for surgical treatment of the inferior turbinates is recommended both in patients with unilateral compensatory hypertrophy related to nasal septum deviation, and in those with chronic bilateral hypertrophy.

Diagnosis

5

The most important step in medicine and surgery is the diagnosis: in this concern, the diagnosis has to be functional and aesthetic.

Computed tomography (CT) of the paranasal sinuses has to be considered as an essential step before taking the decision of a possible nasal surgery (Box 5.1 and Fig. 5.1).

Even when the reasons for surgery are merely aesthetic, CT scanning is necessary for the following reasons:

• of the 80% of the population suffering from respiratory diseases, 30%

Box 5.1 What CT scans show

1. The septum in all of its parts
2. The inferior turbinate with possible hypertrophy
3. The middle turbinate with possible polypoid alterations or bullous conchae
4. The maxillary sinuses with mucosal alterations, sinusitis and polyposis
5. The meatal orifices, communication foramens between nose and sinuses. Serious sinusitis or polyposis may obstruct the orifices, thus triggering increasingly critical diseases
6. The ethmoid and sphenoid sinuses, often affected by inflammatory processes
7. Congenital malformations and abnormalities
8. Expanding tumoral processes

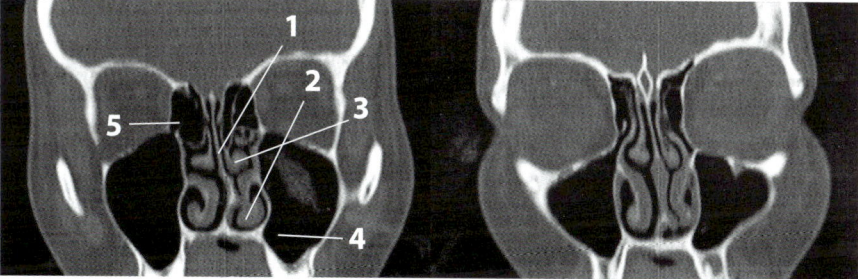

Fig. 5.1 CT scan of the sinuses, frontal section. **1** Nasal septum; **2** inferior turbinates; **3** middle turbinates; **4** maxillary sinuses; **5** meatal ostia

Paolo Gottarelli, *Modified Inferior Turbinoplasty* © Springer-Verlag Italia 2012

have no consciousness of the matter and are asymptomatic, as the inner anatomical alterations are present from infancy and the respiratory memory has not perceived any worsening;

• after reductive rhinoplasty for aesthetic purposes, some previously hidden problems may become evident. The surgeon must therefore feel compelled to avoid such unexpected events;

• a normal skull imaging does not provide satisfactory information because it simultaneously shows an enormous amount of anatomical structures at the caudocranial level, between the nose tip and the ears, which is the actual extension of nose and paranasal sinuses. It should be remembered that the nose communicates with the ears (Eustachian tubes), with the eyes (nasolacrimal duct) and the maxillary, frontal, ethmoidal and sphenoidal sinuses. For these reasons, CT scans are fundamental as they are able to distinguish in subsequent sections all the anatomical structures.

Beyond the detailed assessment of disease extension, some other struc-

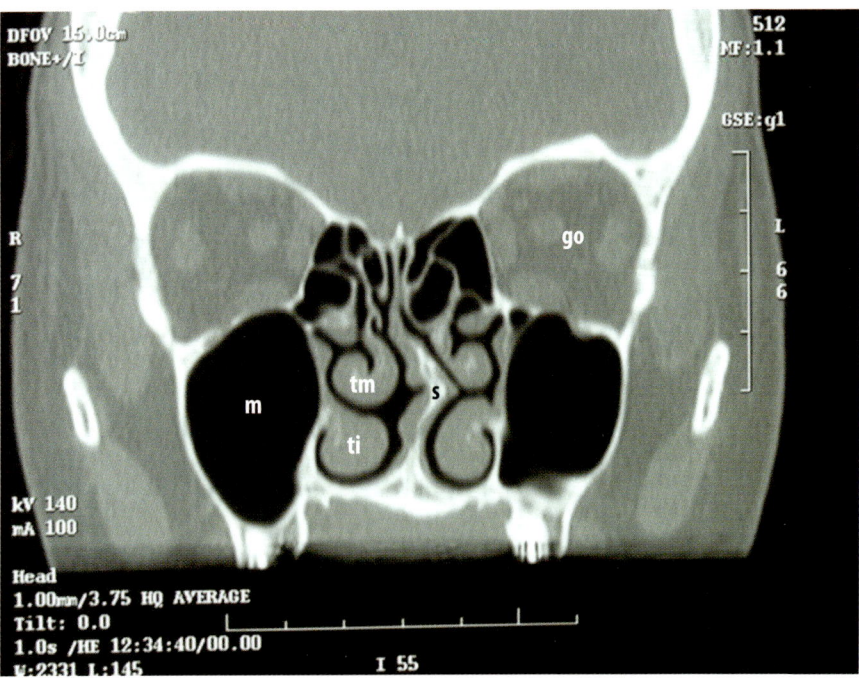

Fig. 5.2 Coronal CT of the paranasal sinuses, which highlights, on the right, the bullous concha; deformation of the right mid-turbinate associated with septal deviation, moved by the abnormal development of the contralateral turbinates towards the opposite side. *go*, ocular bulb; *m*, maxillary sinus; *s*, nasal septum; *tm*, mid-turbinate; *ti*, inferior turbinate

tures accurately detected by a duly performed CT scan are of primary importance for a surgeon (Fig. 5.2).

They consist in:

- the presence of anatomical abnormalities, as the **bullous concha**, of the middle turbinate or the **paradoxical turbinate**;
- the **uncinate process**, a passage leading to the maxillary hiatus below, and the frontal sinus infundibulum above;
- the position of the **anterior ethmoidal artery** crossing the ethmoidal roof with a large number of anatomic variations; this artery must be preserved to prevent orbital bleeding or hematomas;
- the presence of abnormal cells such as **Haller cells** and **Onodi cells**;
- the medial wall of the orbit, the **lamina papyracea**; because of its delicacy, it may be pathologically worn away, thus exposing the fibrous capsule that should remain safeguarded;
- the thickness and position of the **ethmoidal roof**;
- the anatomy of the **sphenoid** and its relation between **internal carotid artery** and **optic nerve**.

How We Attained Modified Inferior Turbinoplasty

6

The inferior turbinates, main organ for respiration and the entire health, are often still treated as if they were anatomic parts not related with the others and almost always with caustic procedures such as laser, electrocautery or even with more advanced radiofrequency therapies: this is a nonsense as well as a deontological issue.

Back in 1951, Howard P. House published on the *Laryngoscope* journal a fundamental trial about the need to evaluate, at any time, not only the external size of the inferior turbinates, but also the possible hypertrophy of the inferior curled bone.

During the 14th International Course of Plastic Surgery at the Clinica Planas in Barcelona, held in June 2004, I had the opportunity of describing once again how the bone portion can become hypertrophic for several reasons. First of all, because of the peculiar conformation of the inferior curled bone, which can be extremely trabeculate so as to make room for the vascular lacunae. Under the centrifugal traction produced by the ingravescent hypertrophy of the soft mucocavernous tissues, the bone increases in volume.

It is essentially an osteogenic mechanical pressure induced by osteodistraction and supported by an increased vascularization. This leads not only to better oxygenation but also to the influx of a greater number of nutrients that enlarge the curled bone size until sometimes it reaches the septum (turbinate-septum clash). The simple dislocation (*out fracture*) of the curled bone cannot guarantee sufficient results, as it does not contribute to achieving a reduction in bone volume, but – as a result of strain trauma – it may lead to further osteofibrous proliferation, capable of nullifying the treatment.

Hence the need to always treat the bone component of the inferior turbinate.

This is the first reason why all the techniques defined as "hot" (laser, electrocautery and radiofrequency) are to be proscribed at all cost. The absurdity of using such techniques is even more evident if we refer to the

Paolo Gottarelli, *Modified Inferior Turbinoplasty* © Springer-Verlag Italia 2012

experiences of dentists and periodontal specialists, proctologists and ophthalmologists.

As a matter of fact, for over two decades, mucogingival hypertrophies
have no longer been treated with those hot techniques, which are responsible for relapses in 100% of cases. The same happens in ophthalmology
when it is necessary to cut the conjunctival mucosa.

Such obvious considerations prompted the need to treat inferior turbinate
hypertrophy using a more scientific and consistent method. The correct
approach to cope with the hypertrophy of all of these three anatomical compartments (lower curled bone, cavernous erectile tissue and mucosal lining)
should be the balanced and uniform dimensional reduction of all three compartments, thus restoring the physiologic ratio.

On this behalf, let us consider the modern approach of surgery towards
hypertrophic breast reduction (gigantomastia). As happens with the inferior
turbinates, breasts are also made of three anatomical compartments: the
gland, the adipose tissue and the skin envelope. Plastic surgeons would never
dream of introducing a needle connected to an acusector into the breast tissue and electrocuting, or to use laser to obtain volume reduction.

In such a case, it has always been clear that the approach must be differ-

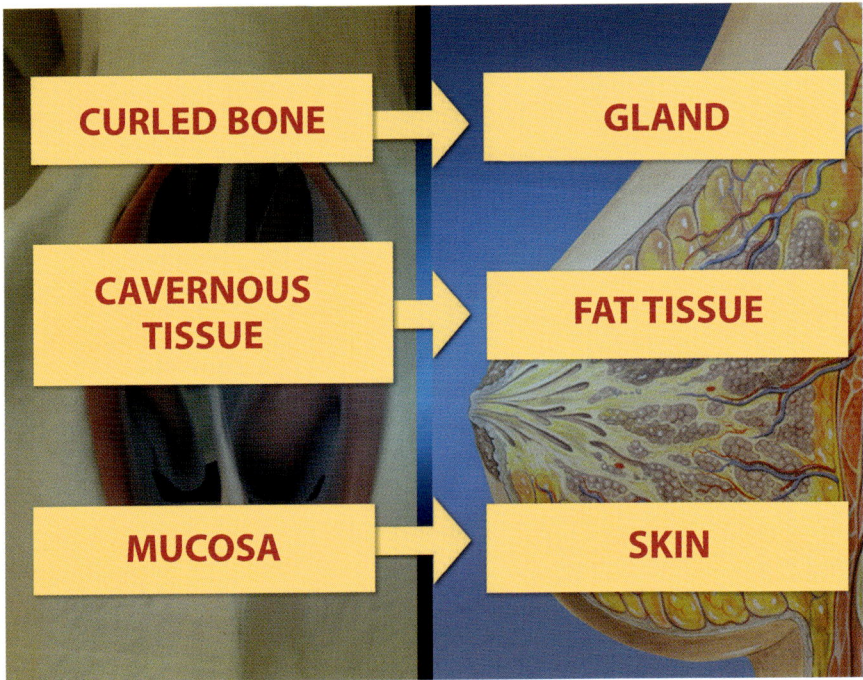

Fig. 6.1 Anatomical structure of the nasal turbinates and the breast

ent. Therefore, why should the intervention on turbinates be different?

The reasons are manifold. The first and most obvious one concerns the anatomical position of the inferior turbinates and the difficulty of being able to correct them completely.

The second reason is represented by common practice and by the fact that the industry has made available to surgeons technical equipments that are very easy to use. But the most critical reason is, as a matter of fact, the lack of a stimulus towards innovation and the well-being of patients.

Another key aspect is the performance of medical and surgical treatments carried out without a correct diagnosis. Too often do we examine patients who have undergone surgical intervention with hot techniques, who unfortunately witness the unavoidable relapses, and present with severe deviations of the nasal septum, sinusitis, reduction of ostium-meatal complex volume, etc., which, as we know very well, are the leading cause of inferior turbinate hypertrophy.

Prior to any intervention, a CT scan is essential to correctly assess all the anatomical structures that define adequate respiration. Lower turbinates showing unmistakable signs of hypertrophy are no accident, but depend on an alteration in uni- or bilateral airflow. In this case, septal deviations represent the main cause of the so-called "compensatory hypertrophy" of one or both inferior turbinates. This is the initial mechanism through which nature tries to limit the overflow of cold air passing through the choana enlarged by the septal deviation (concave portion).

There are also conditions of uni- or bilateral valvular insufficiency, generally caused by trauma or incorrect surgery, that may also change the airflow, thus causing a compensatory hypertrophy through the same pathophysiologic mechanism. A thorough diagnosis should prevent any mistake in surgical treatment choice. These considerations have not only led to the introduction of the modified inferior turbinoplasty (MIT) technique, but also to "Global Rhinoplasty", which represents a rational method to face complex situations and disorders that affect the nose and limit its function by triggering new diseases throughout the respiratory (throat, bronchi and lungs) as well as the myocardial regions.

To sum up, a CT scan of the paranasal sinuses without contrast enhancement should always be performed before surgery, so as to select a surgical approach capable of reshaping the lower turbinates, as happens with hypertrophic breasts. To gain a correct access, it is necessary to use an "open approach", which is the most appropriate method not only to perform MIT, but also to meticulously and predictably perform septoplasty to enlarge the meatal ostia and to restore any anatomical part of a deviated nose.

The New Modified Inferior Turbinoplasty   **7**

Hypertrophy of the inferior turbinates has always represented a serious problem for those involved in nasal surgery.

Back in 1952, the American surgeon Howard P. House drew attention to the fact that hypertrophy of the inferior turbinate was almost always related to the increase in size of the inferior curled bone. Gottarelli later explained this increase in size as caused by two factors: the increased metabolic processes at the expense of the hypertrophic soft tissues caused by hypervascularity and related angiogenesis, and the mechanical factors typical of osteodistraction: since the inferior curled bone is very elastic, trabeculate and also naturally vascularized, the "migration" of the soft parts towards the septal wall creates a kind of traction at the expense of the bone, which starts to stretch and grow.

As a consequence, in order to obtain a correct restoration of the hypertrophic inferior turbinates, it is necessary to also intervene on the curled bone.

In fact, all surgeons recognize the superiority of turbinoplasty compared to simple turbinectomies and to all easier procedures aimed at reducing the soft tissues alone through direct heat application or laser photothermolysis. All these simple and rapid methods show their weak points very soon, within six to twelve months, and sometimes even earlier! This happens because a tissue either resected or treated by thermal stimulation, responds in the medium period by developing secondary hyperplasia. Periodontology, a branch of dentistry that deals with the tooth-supporting apparatus and, in particular, with gum health, has given up many years ago to the use of radiofrequencies and electrocautery for gingival remodeling. This occurred because the recurrence of gingival overgrowth was the rule. Periodontologists have therefore gone back to corrective interventions using cold-cutting scalpels.

The first surgeon who reconciled these needs was Dr. Cottle, who proposed a sort of decompression of the inferior turbinate in its bony and cavernous portion (the tissue lying between the mucosa and the external bone) through a vertical incision at the head of the turbinate.

In 1997, the potential of this technique was further improved, suggesting a longitudinal incision from head to tail of the inferior turbinate, followed by osteocavernous decompression with the reduction of the expanded mucosa. The new method, named modified inferior turbinoplasty (MIT), achieves a total reconstruction through suture flaps made of absorbable material.

This procedure consists of seven distinct surgical steps lasting approximately seven minutes. The big turning point is that, thanks to the precision of the intervention, the onset of cicatricial synechiae (cicatricial tissue between septal wall and turbinate) obstructing the choanae is prevented and the risk of bleeding, in spite of the elimination of endonasal swabs, is virtually abolished.

In the creation of MIT, a crucial role was played by Tebbetts' "open approach", first introduced in Italy by Gottarelli himself.

Among many opportunities offered by the "open approach", there is the careful control of the deep anatomical structures, such as the inferior turbinate.

However, MIT is also feasible with the "closed" surgical approach, although it is not an advisable practice.

Box 7.1 Anatomy of the intervention

The inferior turbinate is made of three parts, like a fruit:

- curled bone   stone
- cavernous tissue   pulp
- mucosa   peel

For this reason, all anatomical components must be reduced, as happens with MIT.

MIT: 7 steps in 7 minutes

- **Infiltration**
  Using a Carpules® syringe, anaesthetic drugs are locally infused (like dentists do before extraction).
  Duration: 15 seconds.

- **Incision**
  The surgeon incides the turbinate longitudinally.
  Duration: 15 to 30 seconds.

- **Limb lifting**
  The turbinate is "opened" by lifting the cut edges. The bony tissue is therefore exposed.
  Duration: 2 minutes.

- **Reduction of bone hypertrophy**
  The bony portion of the turbinate is sharpened: the size is reduced and the hypertrophy corrected.
  Duration: 2 minutes.

- **Reduction of cavernous tissue hypertrophy**
  Through the incision, the size of the cavernous and spongy tissues covering the bony portion of the turbinate are reduced; lastly, the turbinate size is reduced.
  Duration: 1 minute.

- **Washing**
  The operated area has to be cleaned.
  Duration: 15 seconds.

- **Suture**
  The incision is stitched up using a surgical "hair-sized" thread; the suture is hermetic and continuous, the thread is made of polylactic acid (made of carbohydrates) and therefore absorbable.
  Duration: 2 minutes.

After surgery

The nose should not be blown for 5-7 days following intervention. Conversely, accurate washings with seawater or saline thermal water (3-4 times a day) should be performed. Within a month the patient's conditions will normalize.

Post-traumatic Hump Nose

8

Treatment of the post-traumatic nose is extremely delicate and requires highly professional technical equipment. The first rumor to be debunked is that functional surgery is separated from aesthetic surgery. Nothing could be farther from the truth. Functional surgery can never be separated from aesthetic surgery and speaking of aesthetics is not as appropriate as speaking of shaping or, better, of "eumorphy", which means normal and natural shape.

Surgical treatment is difficult because we face the alteration and displacement of most of the anatomical structures that make up the external and internal nose. The nasal pyramid is often diverted to one side and the tip to the other side, the dorsal line has a scoliotic pattern, the lateral cartilages are partially collapsed, as well as the nose tip cartilage. The dislocation and luxation of the most prominent part of the cartilaginous septum (candle septum) lead to collapse of the tip with an opening in one nostril much wider than the other one. Inside the choana, through an anterior rhinoscopy or a deeper endoscopic examination, we may see the cartilaginous septum and the osteoseptum deviated in one or more points; hypertrophy of a turbinate in case of recent trauma or of both turbinates in chronic cases, will therefore be unavoidable. Many of these patients become slaves and addicted to vasoconstrictor sprays, the only weapon to "deflate" the turbinates stuffed with blood and to receive a little airflow.

Using modified inferior turbinoplasty, this intervention, albeit difficult, has reached levels of high result predictability with no postoperative pain, without the application of swabs and with a short and totally safe hospitalization. The versatility of Global Rhinoplasty and the strength represented by the widespread use of cartilage autografts, capable of supporting and reinforcing the deflected and weakened nose, is the utmost that can be done today to treat the nose. The postoperative dressing with small plasters on the dorsum of the nose, covered by a plastic and stiff material, has to be worn for seven days, the same period as with ordinary rhinoplasty, and this again thanks to small cartilaginous supporting and correcting devices that prevent the cartilage from returning to the previous deviation (elastic memory of the septum).

Subsequently, MIT will be performed, as well as the regularization and the centralization of the pyramid. This last maneuver will also be carried out in the least traumatic and most conservative way and in respect of the anatomy: if the nasal bones are off-axis, they should be mobilized to be straightened, but not too much, so as to avoid the risk of excessively narrowing the back of the nose. All this can be obtained using the method introduced in 1986 by Fernando Ortiz Monasterio.

This is the percutaneous greenstick fracture technique; by using 2 mm micro-osteotomes we can reach our goal without producing the scars and trauma typical of the ordinary 4 mm osteotome. The complete fractures of the nasal bones are less precise and less controllable because of an over-mobilization of the bone. The micro-greenstick-osteotomies are, in fact, incomplete micro-fractures that limit the trauma, providing immediate stability.

We will see at this point how the different stages of MIT follow one another, with the support of clear pictorial images.

MIT, Step by Step

9

In this section, the images on the right side are commented in the text.

The nose is made of two nasal cavities separated on the sagittal plane by the septum, with an osteocartilaginous skeleton covered with periosteum and perichondrium.

Structurally, four walls are identified:

- **upper wall** or vault, formed by nasal bones, frontal bone and ethmoid; through the ethmoid cribrate lamina, the olfactory bundles originating from the olfactory bulb enter into the nose;
- **lower wall** or floor, formed by the horizontal plate of palatine bone and by the palatine process of the maxillary bone, which separates the nose from the mouth;
- **medial wall**, or septum, formed (in the antero-posterior direction) by the septal quadrangular cartilage, ethmoid perpendicular lamina, vomer and, below, by the nasal crest of the maxilla and palatine process;
- **side wall**, which consists in the superior and medial turbinates, ethmoid portions, inferior turbinate; moreover, the wall is also formed by the frontal process of the maxilla and by the vertical plate of the palatine. Sometimes there is also the supreme turbinate of Santorini, above the superior turbinate.

The bony protrusions of the **turbinates** run parallel between them and form many meati communicating with the nasal fossae, where the ways out of the paranasal sinuses are: in the upper meatus, the narrowest one, the posterior ethmoid cells drain; in the middle meatus, the largest one, the anterior ethmoid cells, the frontal and the maxillary sinuses drain. These orifices are located in the semilunar hiatus, a groove in the dorsal concavity limited anteriorly by the uncinate process and posteriorly by the ethmoidal bulla; in the inferior meatus drains the nasolacrimal duct.

The nose can be divided into an outer and an inner structure. The balance between these two structures is essential for good respiration. For this reason, the inferior turbinates must always be evaluated in advance even in case of possible aesthetic surgery.

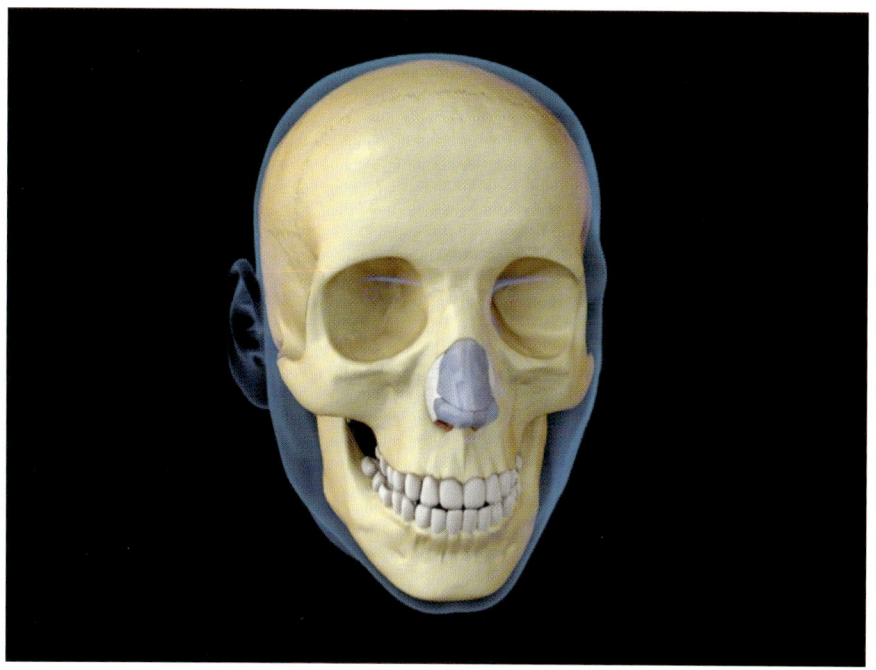

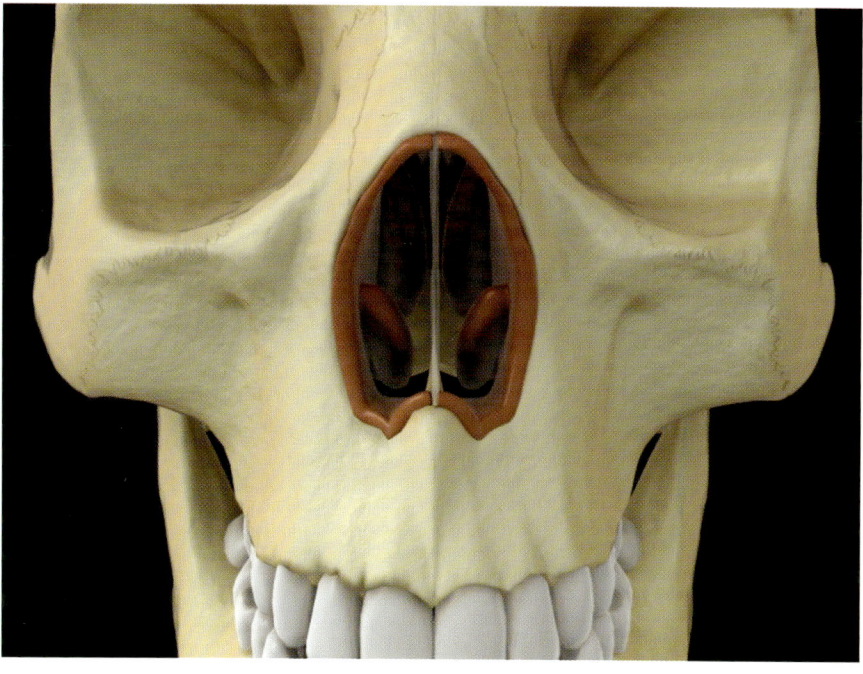

ANATOMY

1. Superior turbinate.

The medial expansion of the ethmoid has a rudimental development in human beings, barely detected under the mucosal lining. It shows a nearly horizontal development and the tail reaches the superior edge of the choana. On its medial surface lies a portion of the olfactory area, which has a peculiar yellow-brownish appearance (*locus luteus*).

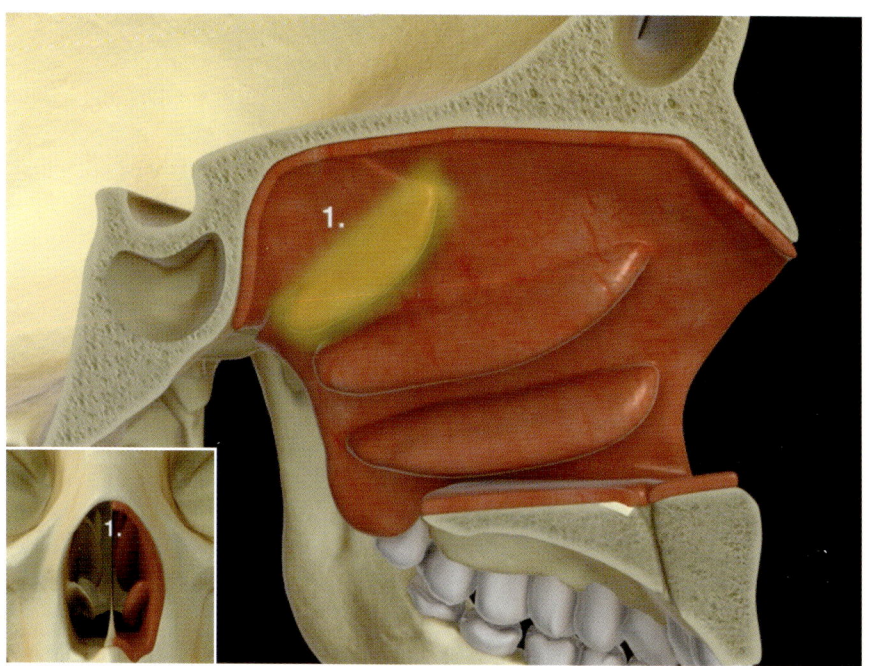

2. Middle turbinate.

It is an ethmoidal, triangular-shaped apophysis, with an anterior basis and a posterior vertex. In the antero-posterior direction, it initially takes an oblique direction, then a horizontal one.

The **medial face** is convex, while the **lateral face** is concave and hides the middle meatal structure.

The **medial lamina,** anteriorly inserted at the basicranium, is covered by the olfactory mucosa and crossed by olfactory nerve fibers. On the rear, instead, the turbinate is loosely anchored to the ethmoid, and only its posterior end is attached to the lateral wall of the nose.

With its **lateral edge** it is attached to the upright branch of the superior maxilla. The **inferior edge** is thick and twisted, and gives rise to the concal sinus (*Zuckerkandl*), sometimes divided into compartments by thin vertical humps. The **anterior end** is a rounded bulge (operculum), separated from the nose wall by a narrow cleft. A small hump (*agger nasi*) starts from the anterior end and extends downwards and frontwards. The head can be pneumatized to varying degrees in 5-10% of individuals (*concha bullosa*), a finding first described by Santorinus (1724) and reported with evidences by Zuckerkandl (1893). Often unilateral, it may sometimes reach a considerable size (28 mm), spreading to touch the septum or the inferior turbinate, or grazing the floor of the nasal fossa. In the middle turbinate, the presence has been proved of cystic forms, admirably described by Radoievitch et al. (1959). Already present in the embryo (Kikuchi, 1903), and noticed at all ages, they are lined up with the same mucosa as the ethmoidal cells (Kikuchi, 1903; Harmer, 1903). In very rare cases, meningocele has been reported (O'Brien, 1931). The **back end** (tail) reaches the supero-lateral corner of the choana, approximately 12-14 mm from the tubal ostium.

The **concha bullosa** is an abnormality in middle turbinate development: instead of being a flat bone that limits the middle meatus, i.e. the area where the paranasal sinuses open, favoring the entrance of inhaled air, it takes on a globular shape and blocks the meatus, producing nasal respiratory obstruction, which patients report as "high". Owing to the malfunction of the paranasal sinus orifices, recurrent episodes of sinusitis are frequently reported.

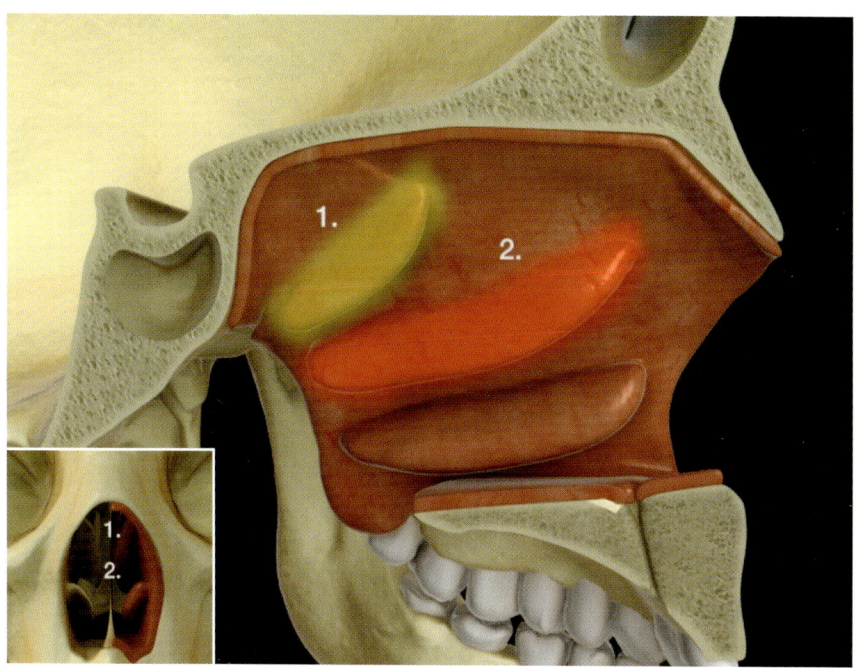

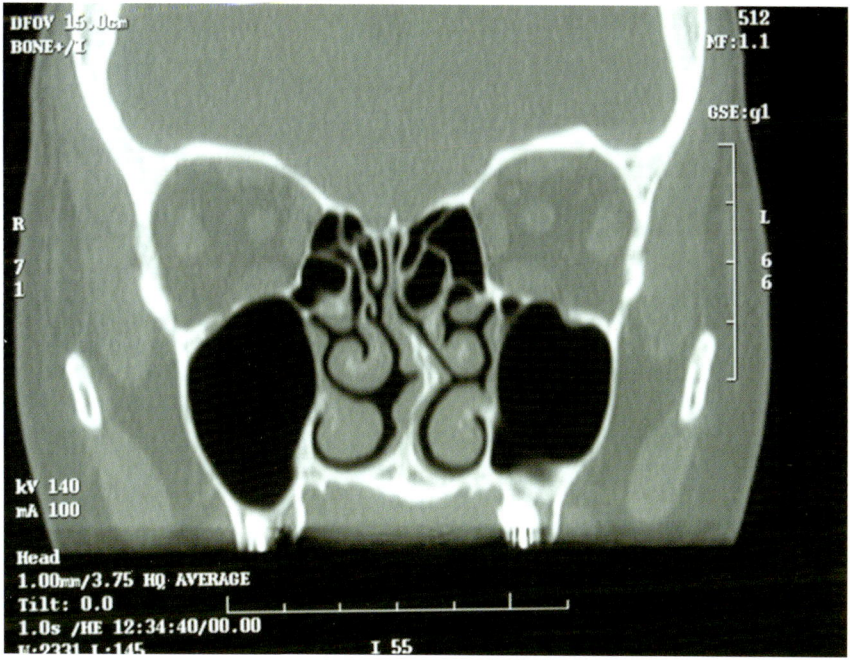

3. Inferior turbinate.

This is an independent, paired, symmetrical and thin bone, folded on itself, sagittally elongated, triangular in shape. In the anterior portion it is slightly oblique downwards and frontwards, and procedes almost horizontally near the floor of the nasal fossa. The rear end, instead, is very sharp.

The inferior turbinate has two free faces, two joint edges, a free edge and two ends.

- **Internal or nasal face**. An oblique ridge divides downwards and backwards this convex face into two sides, superior and inferior. The shape of the curled bone and the amplitude of the meatus depends on the direction (horizontal or oblique) of the superior side. Conversely, the inferior side always has a sagittal trend and shows a surface plagued by irregular bony ridges.
- **External or meatic face**, concave and less bumpy than the nasal face. The shape of the superior (free) margin influences its depth: when it is folded on itself some grooves are formed, becoming areas of stagnant secretions.
- **Joint (anterior and postero-superior) margins**. The superior edge is connected with the upright branch of the superior maxilla. The postero-superior edge has an oblique direction downwards and backwards. It is anteriorly connected with the posterior lip of the lacrimal dacryocyst and posteriorly with the posterior turbinal crest of the palatine bone. The apophyseal system of the superior turbinate is originated from the superior margin and it consists, in the antero-posterior direction, of the lacrimal process (the external face forms, together with the lacrimal dacryocyst of the superior maxilla, the naso-lacrimal duct; the inner face corresponds to the anterior segment of the middle meatus), in the maxillary or auricular process, so called for its peculiar shape resembling a dog's ear, and in the ethmoid process, *trait d'union* with the uncinate process.
- **Free margin**. Considerably thick, it is close (4-5 mm) to the nasal cavity floor.
- **Anterior end (head)**. Next to the piriform ridge (2-3 mm), it is attached with its anterior edge to the upright branch of the maxilla.
- **Posterior end (tail)**. It is located approximately 1 cm from the tubal opening, whose function can be seriously damaged by disorders of the tail.

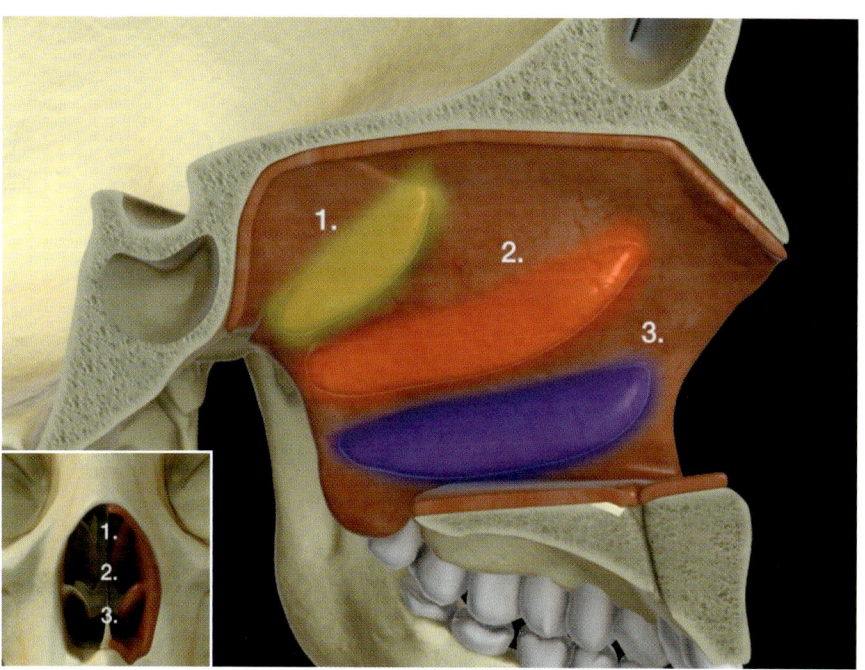

Superior meatus. Poorly developed, it is to be taken into consideration because its anterior portion leads to the orifices of the posterior ethmoidal cells. Its anterior portion contains the **olfactory cleft**, that extends up the upper part, between septum and mid-turbinate, towards the root of the nose. Posteriorly, the superior meatus is narrowed by the anterior wall of the **sphenoid**.

Middle meatus. Limited superiorly and medially by the internal face of the middle curled bone and laterally by the nasal wall, it represents a fundamental cavity from a clinical and surgical viewpoint. It receives the draining orifices of the maxillary sinus, anterior ethmoid and frontal sinus.

Knowledge of the ratio between the lateral wall of the meatic cavity and the adjacent formations is of primary importance: downwards, the maxillary sinus; in the remaining portion the medial wall of the orbit and the dacryocyst. This wall is quite regular in the anterior and posterior portion, while the middle one is crossed by two humps (uncinate process and bulla) and two grooves (uncinate process groove and bulla groove). The two humps, backwards and downwards, are considered by some authors as "rudimentary turbinates" while, according to Mouret's opinion, they are *inversés et éversés* turbinates, i.e. their meatus is located up and backwards instead of being down and frontwards. From this viewpoint, the uncinate process groove represents the meatus of the same process, while the groove of the bulla constitutes the meatus of the bulla itself.

The **uncinate process** (**unciform apophysis**) is a thin bony scimitar-shaped lamella. It adheres to the lateral wall only in correspondence to the antero-superior (ethmoidal) and postero-inferior (maxillary) ends. The mid-portion (body) may have a different morphology and direction. The inferior end crosses the main orifice of the maxillary sinus and sends three extensions: inferior, towards the inferior turbinate; posterior, to the palatine bone; postero-superior, to the bulla. The bounded surfaces may lack a bony wall.

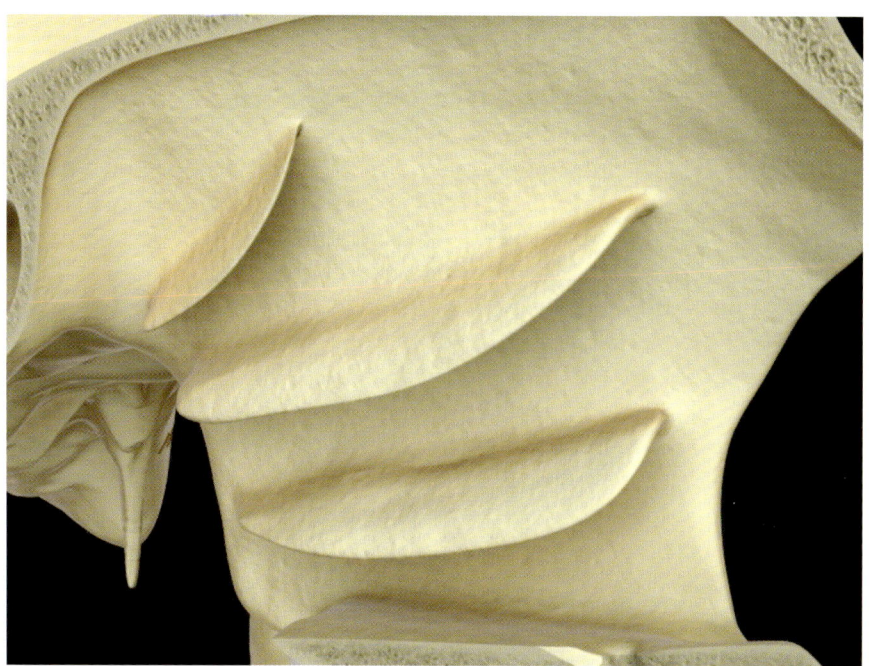

ANATOMY

Inferior meatus. It is the area between the concave face (external or meatal) of the inferior turbinate and the nasal wall. The latter consists of three separate structures: the inner face of the upright branch of the superior maxilla (anterior third); the inner portion of the maxillary sinus (middle third) and the palatine bone (posterior third). In the anterior third the nasolacrimal duct opens, while the boundary between the maxillary and the palatine is marked by a hiatus, made of a thin bony lamina: the auricular apophysis, *locus minoris resistentiae*, of the maxillary sinus wall.

The amplitude of the meatal cavity varies greatly, depending on whether the inferior turbinate is flattened or rounded.

As a general rule, we will have in the first case a long curled bone, a narrowed nasal concha and a reduced meatus; in the second case, the curled bone will look short, the nasal concha will be grooved with very marked humps and the meatus will be large with a reduced-sized maxillary sinus.

The increased vascularity caused by mucocavernous hypertrophy creates a force (osteodistraction) capable of dragging the curled bone towards the septum, even thanks to an accelerated osteogenesis, increased by metabolic processes.

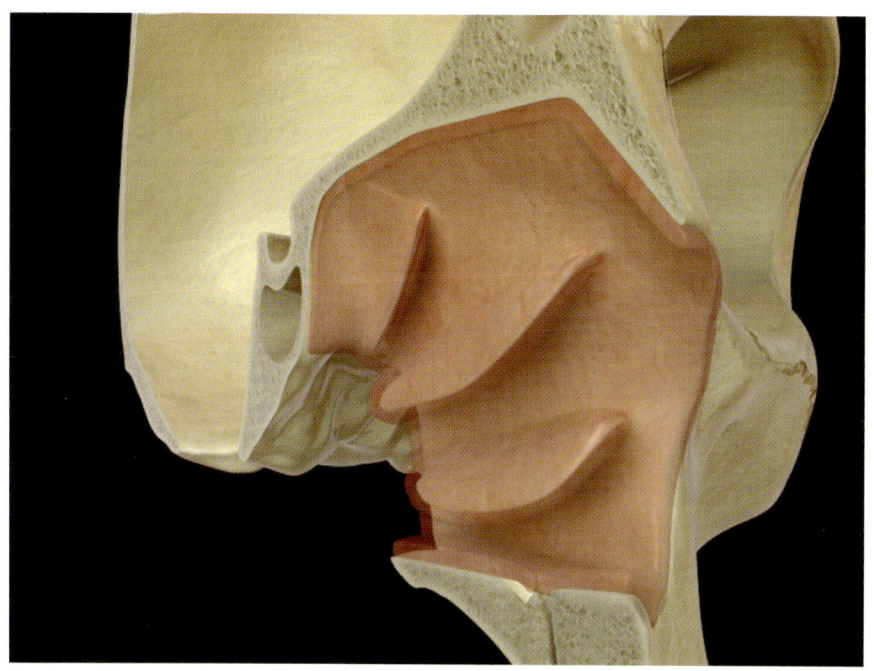

The factors responsible for turbinate disorders are manifold: the most common pathological conditions are allergic, vasomotor or drug-related disorders, together with the so-called compensatory hypertrophy, which gradually develops on the opposite side of the septal deviation at the expense of the bony, vascular and glandular tissues of the nose. The connected causal element is chronic "irritative" stimuli of different nature: allergic, nervous, chemical, thermal, mechanical and pharmacological reasons.

Therefore, from a histopathological viewpoint, hypertrophic-hyperplastic disorders of increasing severity and decreasing reversibility develop. Actual hypertrophy is still a physiological response, characterized by glandular hyperactivity, sinusoid dilatation and stromal cell hypertrophy. This stage is characterized by the possibility of reducing swelling after local vasoconstrictor application.

In the next stage (hyperplasia) some structural alterations develop, confirming the irreversible pathological frame: thickening of the epithelial layer, cellular infiltration of the real tunica, neoformation of blood vessels, proliferation and myxoid degeneration of connective tissue stroma, hypertrophy of the curled bone, mostly in the inferior turbinate.

CT imaging (*below left*) shows hypertrophy of the right inferior curled bone.

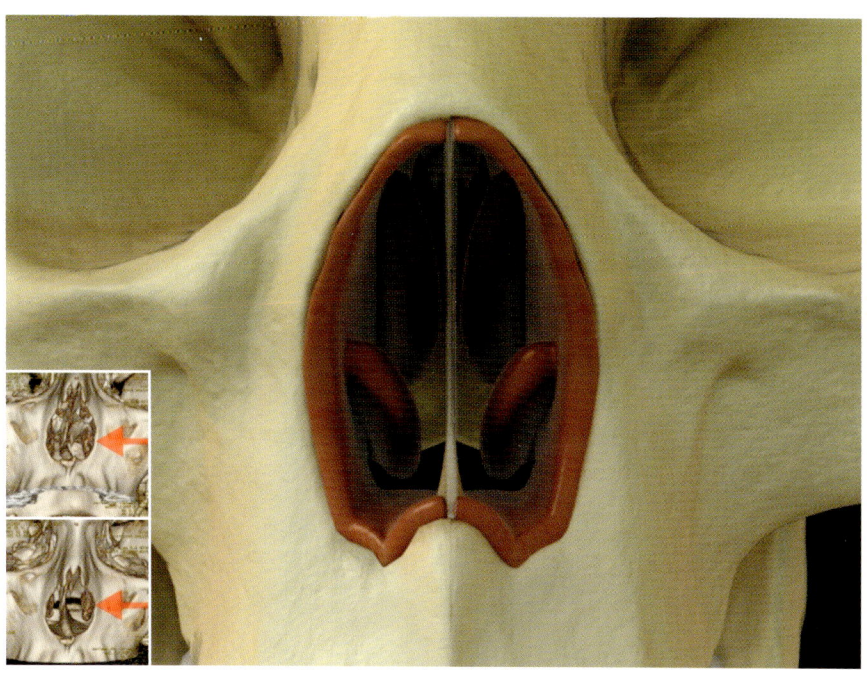

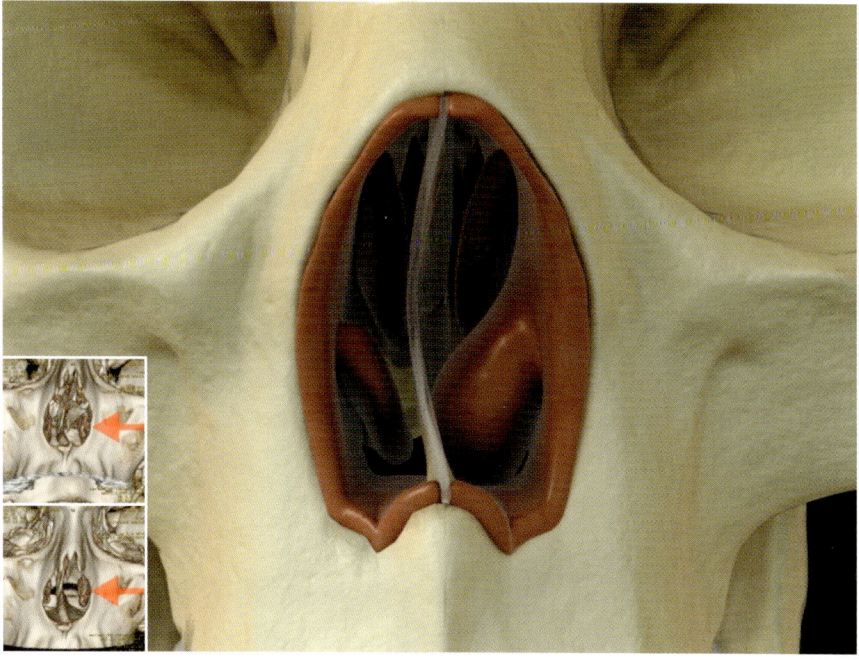

PATHOLOGY

Compensatory hypertrophy: CT imaging with evidence of the hypertrophic curled bone.

These structural changes can be located above all at the rear end of the turbinate (in particular the inferior curled bone), leading to the so-called *morular degeneration* of the turbinate tail. This disease is responsible for very different symptoms: nasal stenosis, mostly during expiration, sleep discomfort, mucopurulent discharge in the nasopharynx, auditory disorders, dry throat, pharyngeal tenesmus, as well as symptoms reflected by the nearby structures.

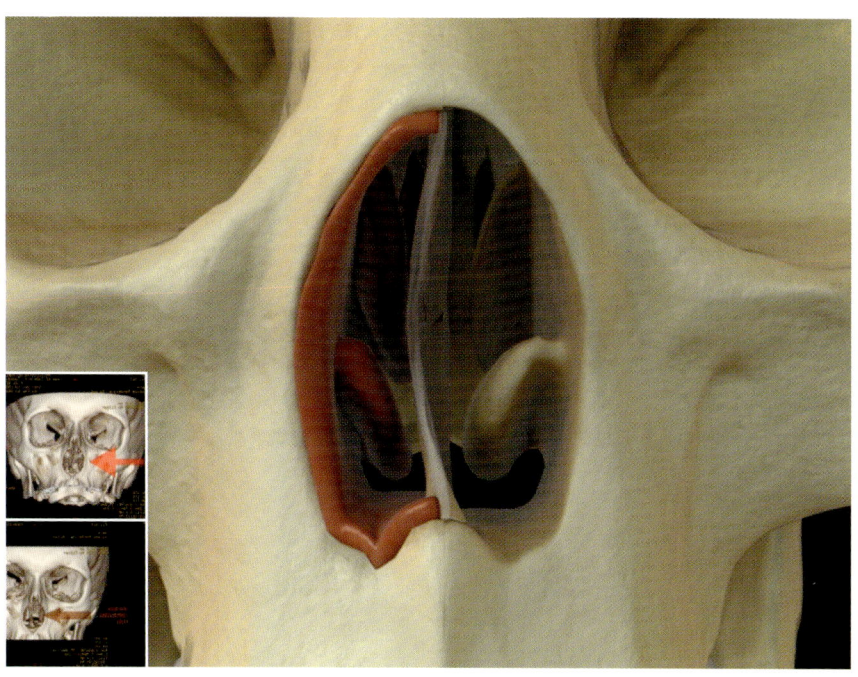

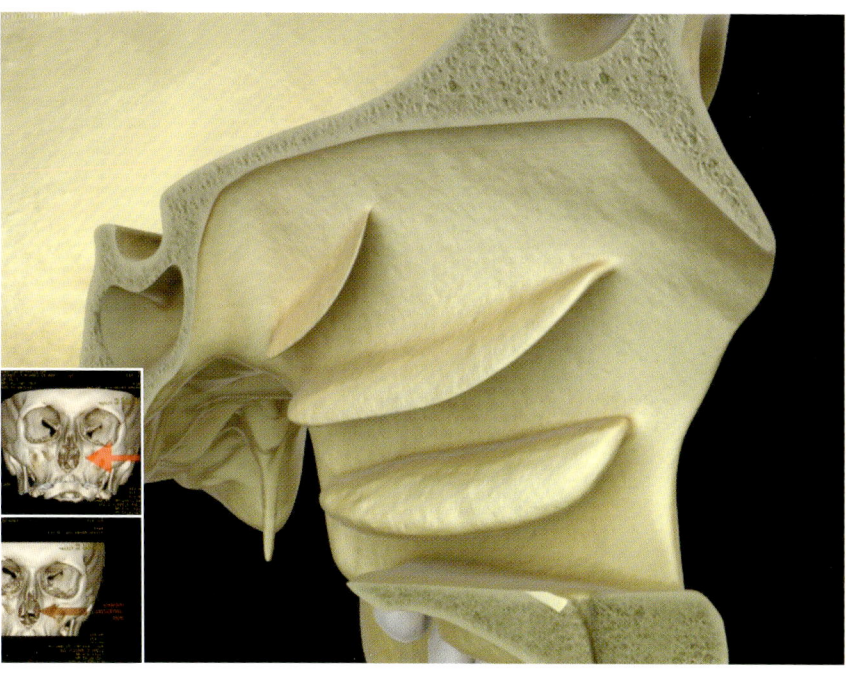

PATHOLOGY

The inferior turbinate, largely made of erectile tissue, is the most frequently involved structure. However, there is also evidence of these formations in the middle turbinate at the rear end of the septum. These changes in turbinate size modify the volume and shape of the nasal cavities with a lumen reduction resulting in a significant increase in nasal resistance (law of Blasius).

Compensatory hypertrophy: CT imaging (*above and below left*) with evidence of hypertrophic curled bone.

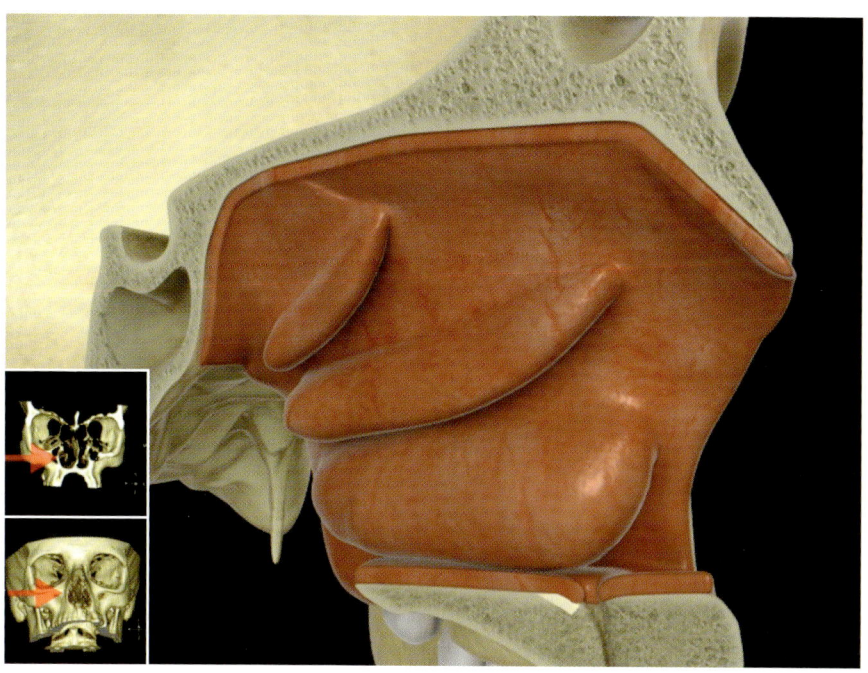

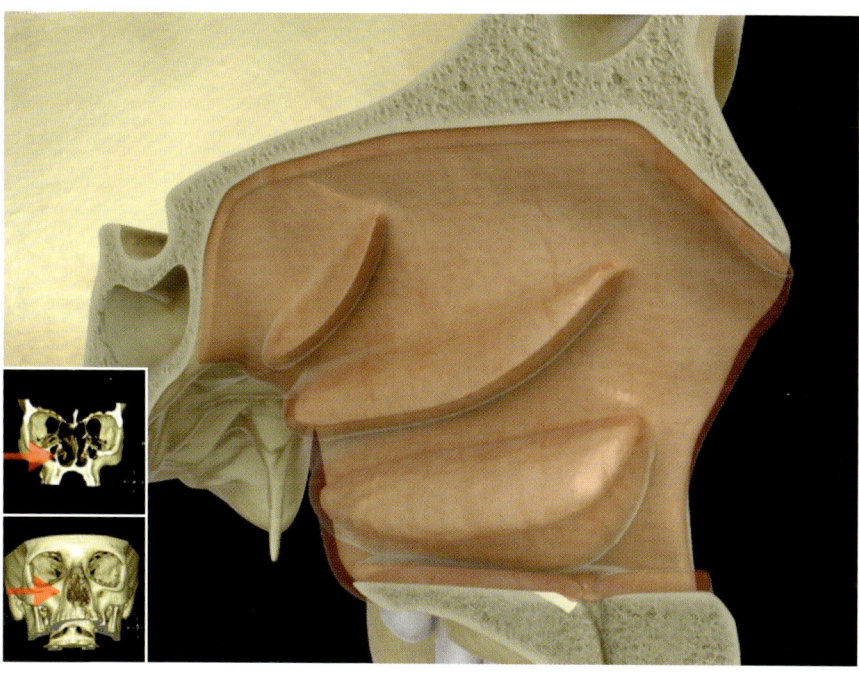

The inferior turbinates, whose skeleton is made of an independent little bone, are the largest and longest nasal turbinates (4-5 cm), with a triangular oblong shape and an anterior base corresponding to the head of the turbinate, located few millimeters away from the nostril; the posterior apex or tail of the turbinate is located 1 cm away from the opening of the Eustachian tubes.

The respiratory portion of the nasal fossae, along with large sections of the olfactory structure, is lined with a smooth, pink-colored mucosa, 2 mm thick at septal level. It becomes thicker, up to 5 mm, at the inferior turbinate level, rich in **cavernous or erectile tissue**, especially at the head and tail levels.

The physico-chemical stimulation of the nasal mucosa is expressed in a reflected way, at the nose level, with circulatory changes, especially in the erectile tissue of the turbinate, accompanied by changes in the lumen of the nasal fossae and by increase in glandular secretion, mainly serous and mucous. At the same time, the reflex decreases the amplitude and rhythm of the respiratory system; the air can remain sufficiently in touch with the surface of the nasal mucosa and is conditioned in temperature, humidity and purity.

The cavernous tissues are particularly important for the **vasomotor reactions**. Since this tissue is mainly present at the inferior turbinate level, these structures are essential for correct breathing.

Temperature and level of humidity of inspired air are emblematic variables in the characterization of inferior turbinate vasomotor reflex: cold air causes congestion of the cavernous spaces, as well as excessively hot and dry air. On the other hand, hot and moist air causes decongestion of the inferior turbinate. The mechanical or chemical stimulation of the nasal mucosa leads to an increased secretion of serous, particularly fluid material. The marked vasomotor and secretory reflexes of the nasal mucosa are closely related and play a very important role in nose defense. This high reactivity can exceed the limits, going from physiological to pathological, in the so-called neurodegenerative nasal syndromes, such as hypertrophic inferior turbinate vasomotor rhinitis.

It is therefore essential to reduce all three anatomical components of the inferior turbinates as suggested by the MIT method.

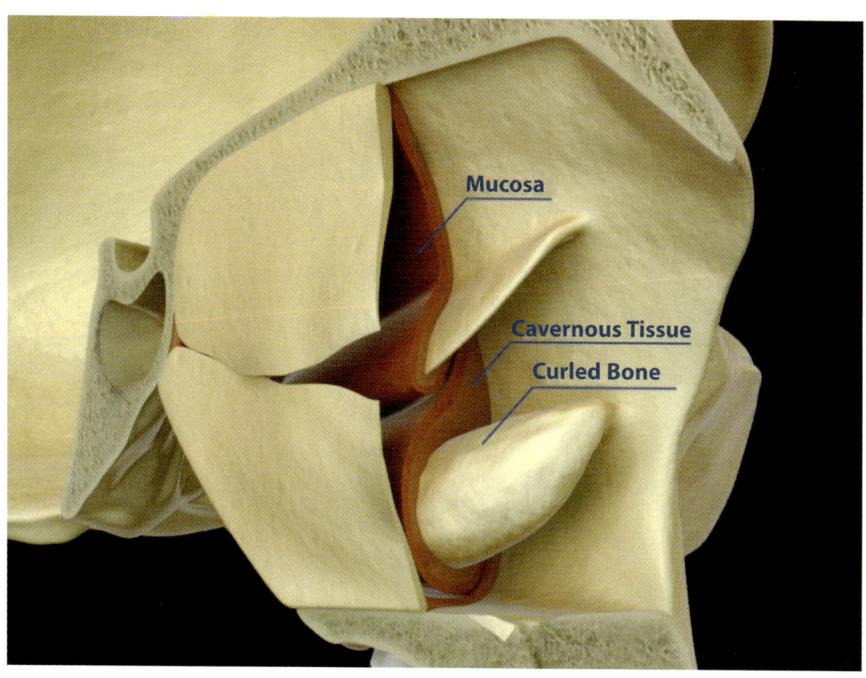

MIT offers the possibility to be free from vasoconstrictor addiction, without the use of "hot" techniques such as laser, radiofrequency and diathermo-electrocoagulation (DEC), through a simple, completely painless operation without the use of swabs.

More than twenty years ago dentists, periodontists, proctologists and ophthalmologists have stopped cutting mucous membranes with "hot" techniques, both because of the inevitable relapses and of the tissue alterations induced by these interventions. Furthermore, "hot" techniques have proved to be ineffective against bone hypertrophy.

DEC is one of the so-called "hot" techniques that must not be considered as resolutive in the treatment of osteo-mucocavernous hypertrophy of the inferior turbinate.

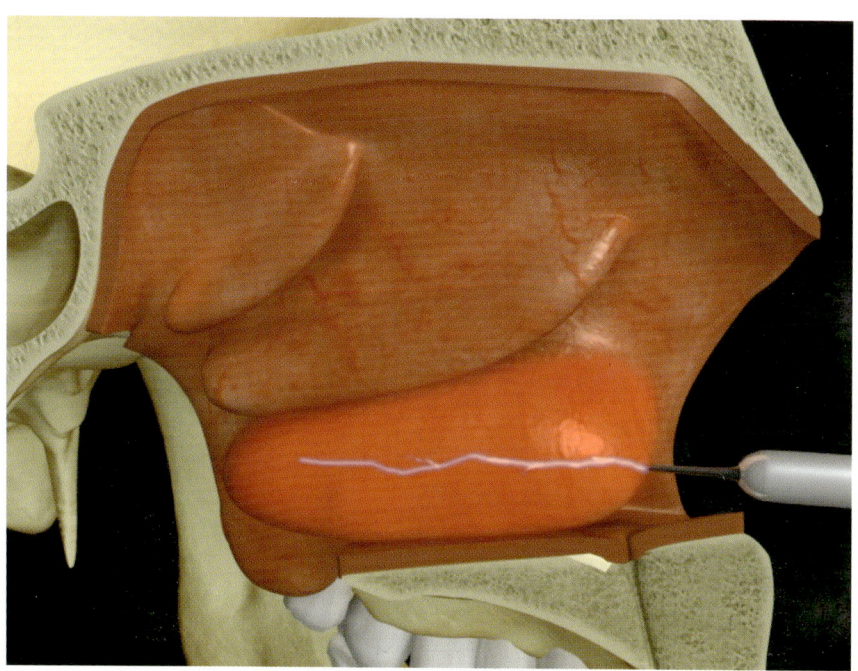

Open rhinoplasty is performed through a small cut in the middle of the columella that will be almost unrecognizable upon complete recovery. Through the columellar incision, all structures are exposed: alar and triangular cartilages, nasal valve, septum and dorsal bone.

The surgeon is thus able to examine and assess any abnormality in shape, asymmetry or structural alteration to be corrected with the highest accuracy. Any suture and graft can be performed with extreme precision.

In order to avoid any scar, surgeons perform particular cuttings with different shapes, according to the surgeons who developed the techniques. The suture is made with thin wires and after 2-3 weeks the scar is almost imperceptible and becomes virtually invisible upon complete recovery.

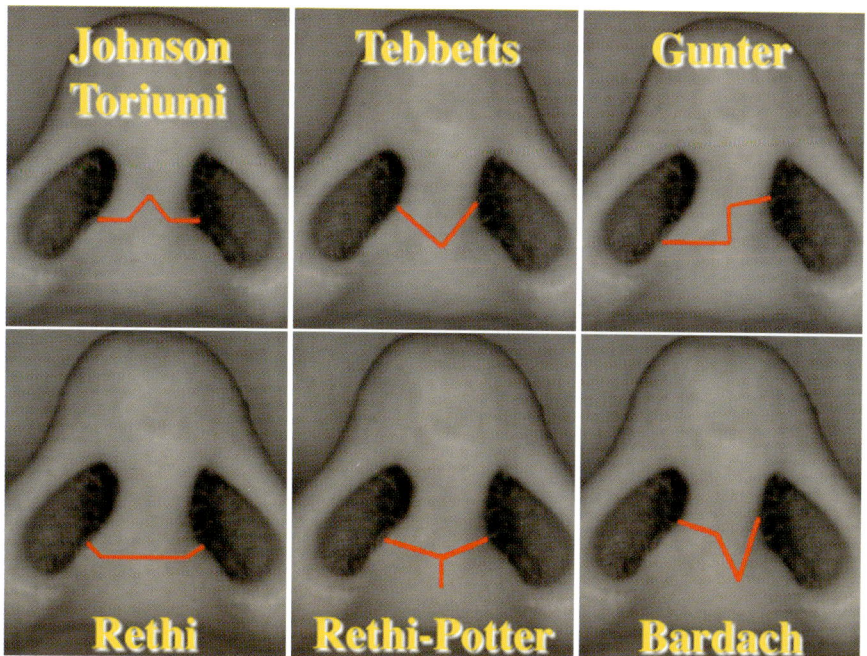

The first step in MIT is suggested by the need to operate in a bloodless field as much as possible; since the cavernous tissue is very rich in blood, it is essential to follow this preliminary step.

- The first reason is to reach an adequate vasoconstriction that allows us to work in a bloodless field.
- The second reason is the creation of an hydrodissection between the soft tissues and the inferior curled bone of the turbinate.
- The third reason is that the injected fluid amplifies the turbinate volume and solidifies it, thus highlighting the exact point for the longitudinal incision.

Infiltration is performed by using a dental Carpules® syringe with a 27-gauge, 35-mm needle. A cartridge is inserted into a dental-type syringe, with a solution of mepivacaine 1:100,000 with epinephrine.

Infusion is carried out by inserting the needle into the head of the turbinate, first superficially as to blanch the mucosa, then reaching the bony level of head, body and tail of the turbinate.

A 1.8 mL cartridge is sufficient to achieve the desired result. It is recommended to wait few minutes during which additional washings of cartilaginous septum will be performed, evacuating small hematomas formed between the two mucosal layers. As a matter of fact, it must be remembered that inferior turbinoplasty should always be performed after spur and deviation correction. This is necessary to take advantage of the widest working area inside the choana, always taking into consideration that in order to solve the patient's respiratory disease, it is absolutely necessary to remove all the causes originating turbinate hypertrophy. At this point, after few minutes, a n. 14 nasogastric probe is inserted, connected to an aspirator that is positioned in the nasopharynx through the other nasal opening. This simple maneuver allows to work more easily in an operating area free from blood, but also from the solution (saline) with which choanae and turbinate are continuously irrigated.

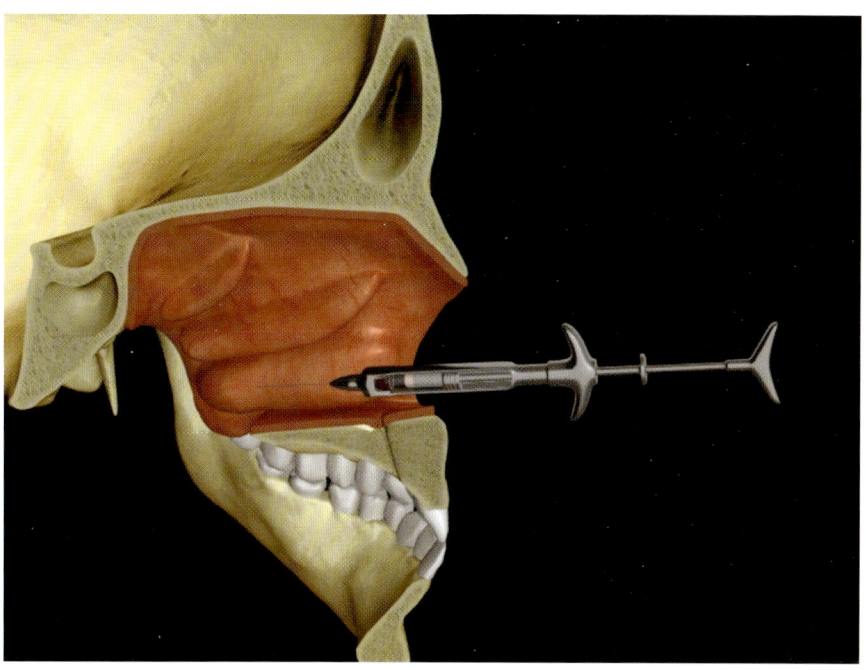

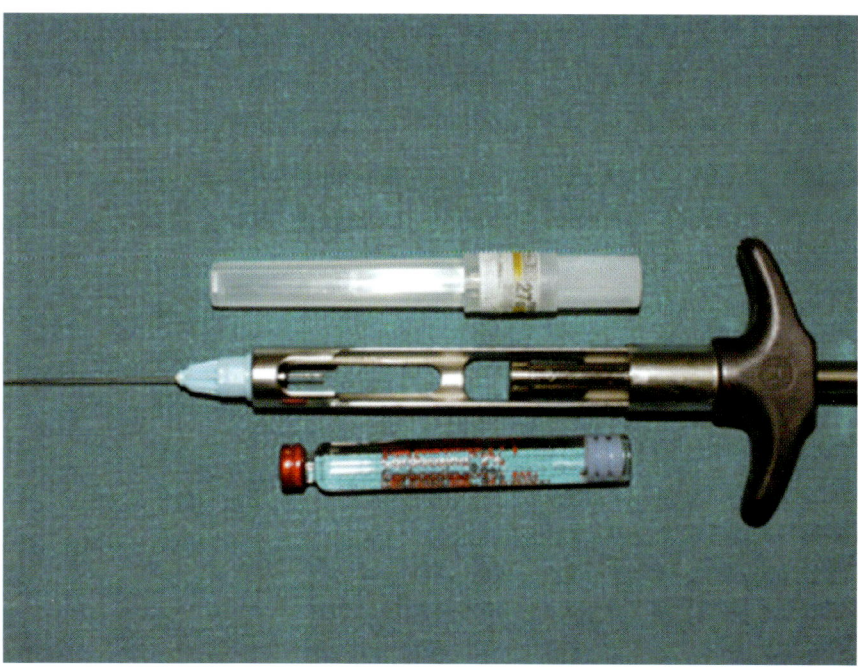

Once the first step of MIT is completed, the incision is performed, using a Bard-Parker handle blade, size 15, Aesculap Inc.

The incision should be carried out longitudinally from the body towards the head of the inferior turbinate, taking care to remain along the midline. The blade must be sunk to the periosteum and then brought up to the head of the turbinate.

Great attention must be paid when the cut is approaching the head of the turbinate as there are many anatomical variations and one of the two edges to be lifted could be completely detached. In this unfortunate case, without being discouraged, the nasopharynx flap head must be recovered and immediately sutured to the contralateral one. It is advisable to practice at least two stitches in Vicryl 5/0 to better stabilize the flaps on the head of the turbinate. Once this stabilization is fulfilled, the intervention can continue regularly.

The incision of the turbinate tail will only be performed after sufficiently detaching the soft tissues from the bone: in this case, it is better to continue the separation of the flaps using angled scissors that, where the turbinate tapers off, allow for a safe incision.

By accurately performing the first and second steps of MIT, as described above, one can observe the gaping of the arteriola only in 0.5% of the cases. When this occurs, it is recommended to coagulate the vessel with an acu-sector using a Colorado tip with 30° angulation.

A new irrigation with saline is then practiced and the next step of detachment and lifting of the two mucocavernous flaps can be performed.

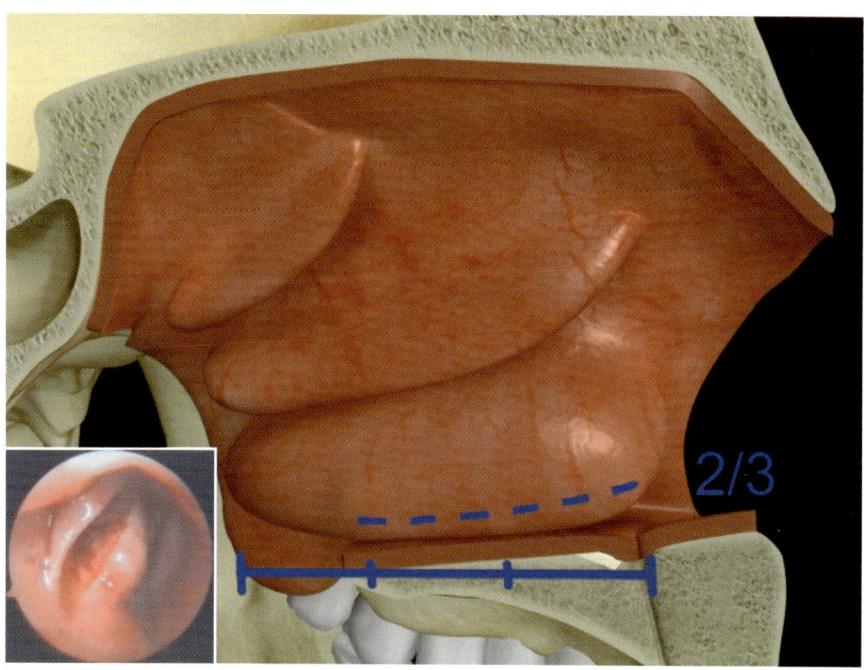

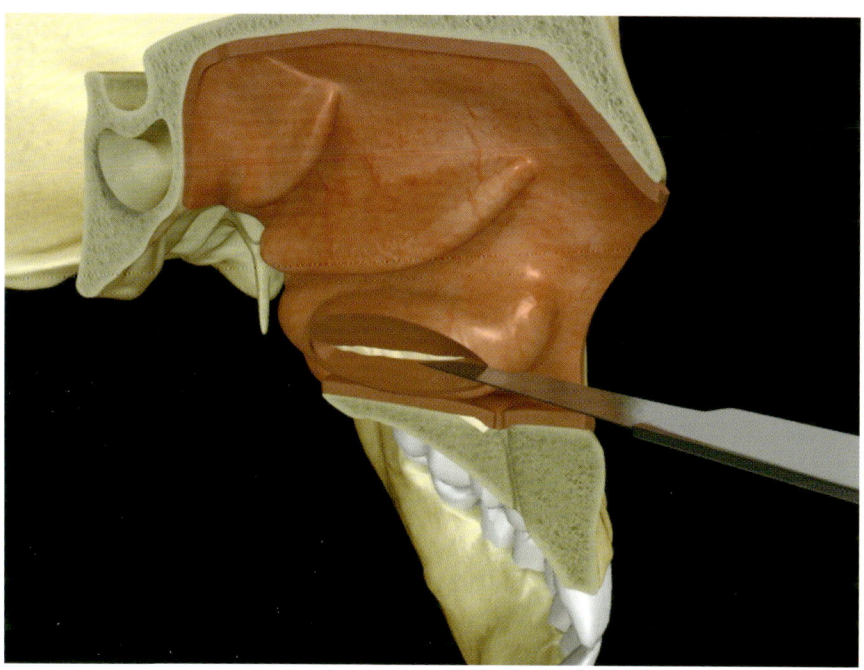

This third step is crucial to be able to perform the following reduction of the underlying hypertrophied curled bone and have a suitable sliding of the mucocavernous tissue carrying out a correct suture. By using the access way created through the incision, and using a particularly thin periosteotome, the soft portion of the bone is gently separated, starting from the head up to the body of the turbinate. Once the body is detached, even laterally, detachment continues along the midline, creating a tunnel where the angled scissors will pass; this will allow for enlargement of the incision along the tail of the turbinate without risking laceration of the mucosa.

Now the detachment can free the curled bone completely from the soft parts, thus facilitating the subsequent removal of bony excess. Even in this step, washings with saline solution should be repeatedly performed.

Instruments used to perform MIT correctly.

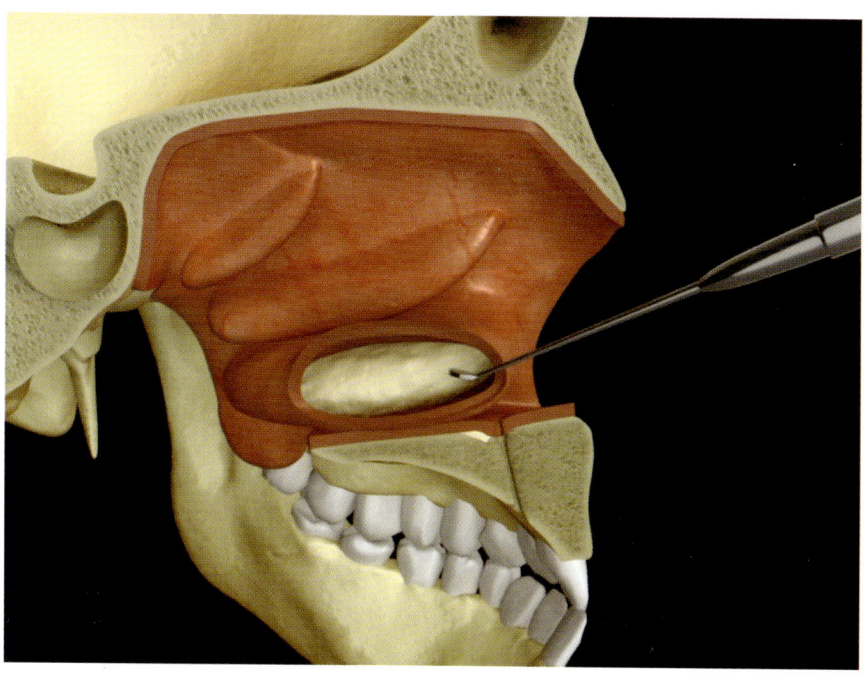

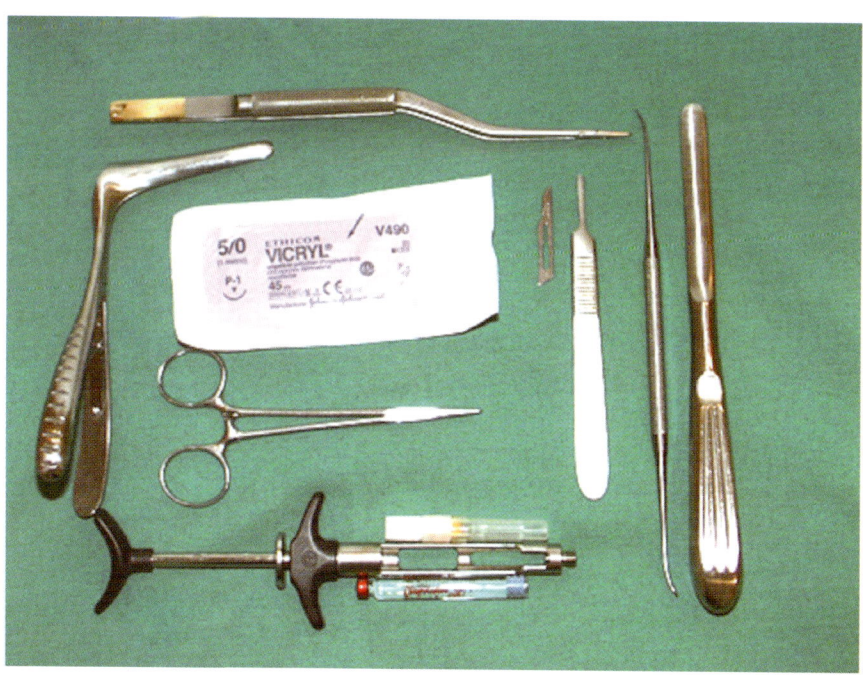

This fourth step of turbinoplasty is of primary importance: it must be known that the turbinate bone gets consistently hypertrophic with soft tissue hypertrophy; therefore, if a good reduction of the inferior turbinate is to be obtained, the soft tissues must not be the only ones to be cauterized.

Moreover, some surgeons maintain that dislocation (out-fracture) of the turbinate may be sufficient, because the air will have more space to get in simply by moving the turbinate externally. This maneuver is certainly very useful as a palliative, but the fibrotic repair of the out-fracture will soon cause a new increase in volume, partially nullifying the result. All this will be facilitated by the increased residual presence of blood (mucocavernous hypertrophy) frequently occurring after laser, radiofrequency and electro-cautery treatment.

This is why, once the curled bone is entirely isolated, partial removal will be performed using nippers, simply through the careful and gentle use of a Freer detacher. It is sufficient to leave a moderate amount of bone as soft tissue support, while a complete removal of the inferior curled bone could cause a soft tissue gaping during respiration. This situation is to be avoided at all costs.

A simple CT scan confirms how and how much the curled bone is hypertrophied, perfectly highlighting what has occurred inside the inferior turbinate. Back in 1952, the *Laryngoscope* magazine issued a study by Howard P. House on the need to reduce the turbinate, bony structure included. Almost 60 years later it is not difficult to notice that the majority of surgeons, instead of performing turbinoplasty correctly, limit to "scorching" the soft tissues with different devices. This way, reductions of the soft parts are performed separately, without removing the causes that have led to turbinate hypertrophy.

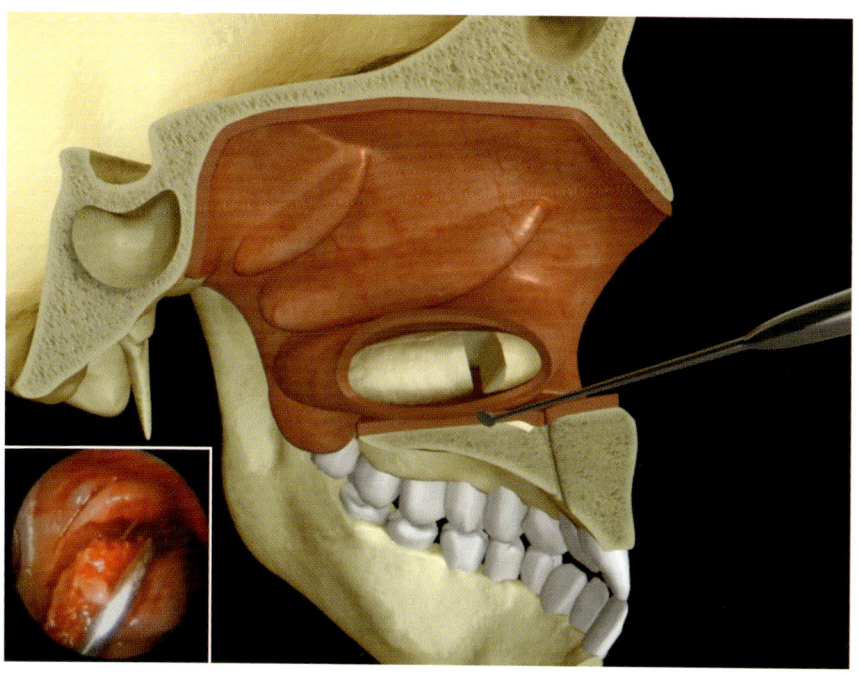

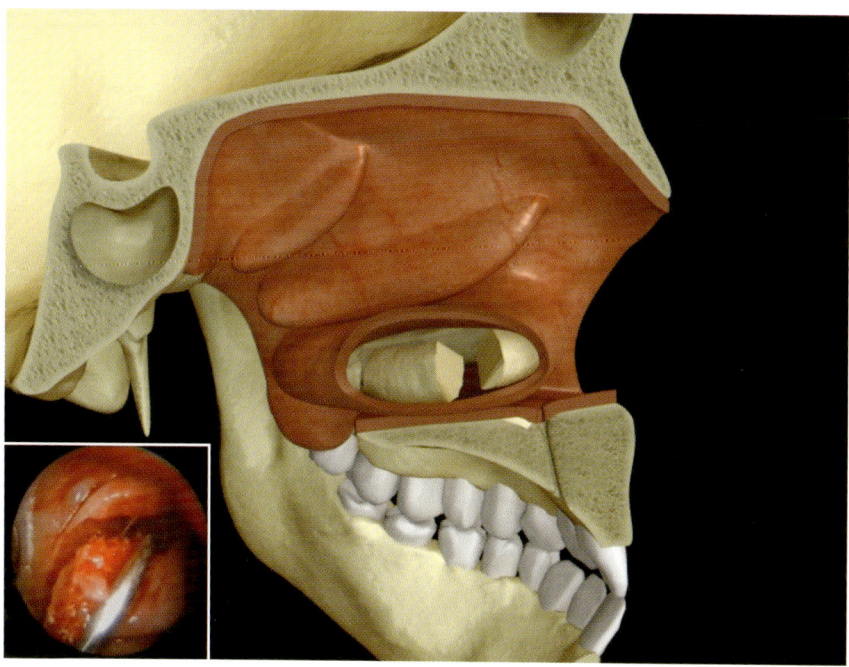

Removal of fragments of the surgically reduced hypertrophic curled bone.

When removing the fragments of the curled bone, it is necessary to leave a moderate amount of bone as support for the soft parts: the risk of a total ablation of the curled bone could cause a gaping of the soft parts during breathing.

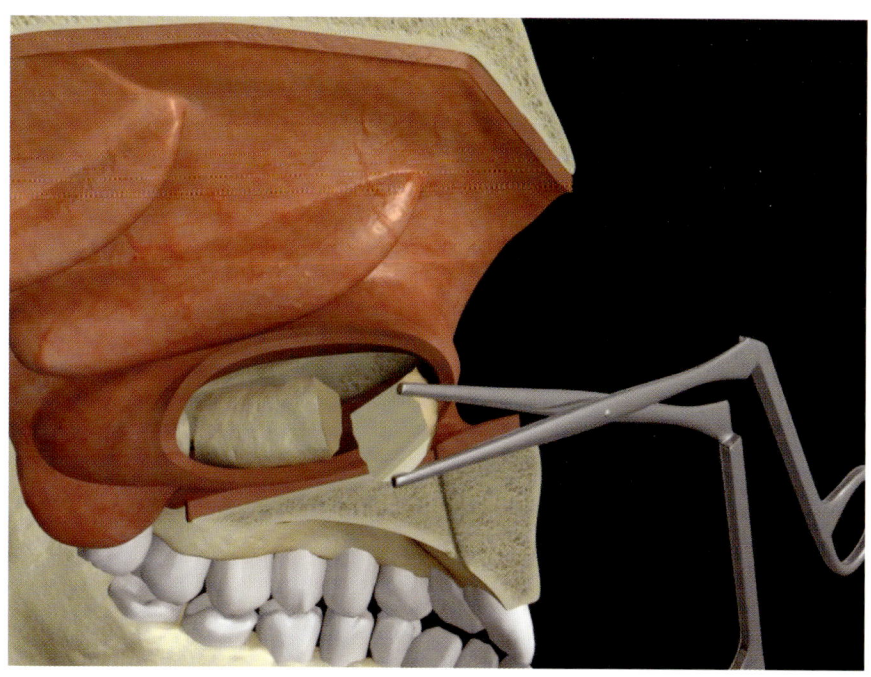

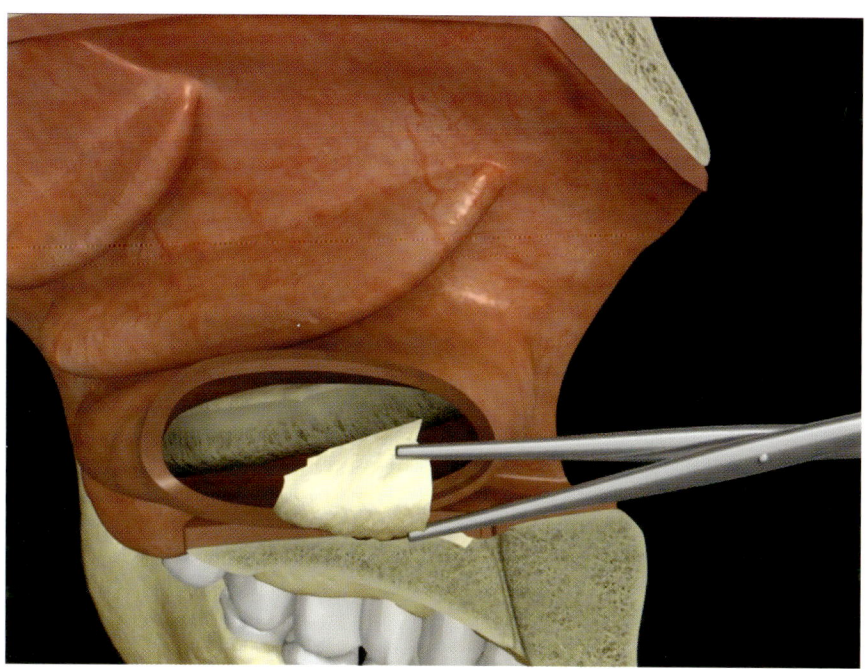

At this point, the inferior turbinate can be compared to the stone of a fruit: a cherry that has enlarged to the size of an apricot.

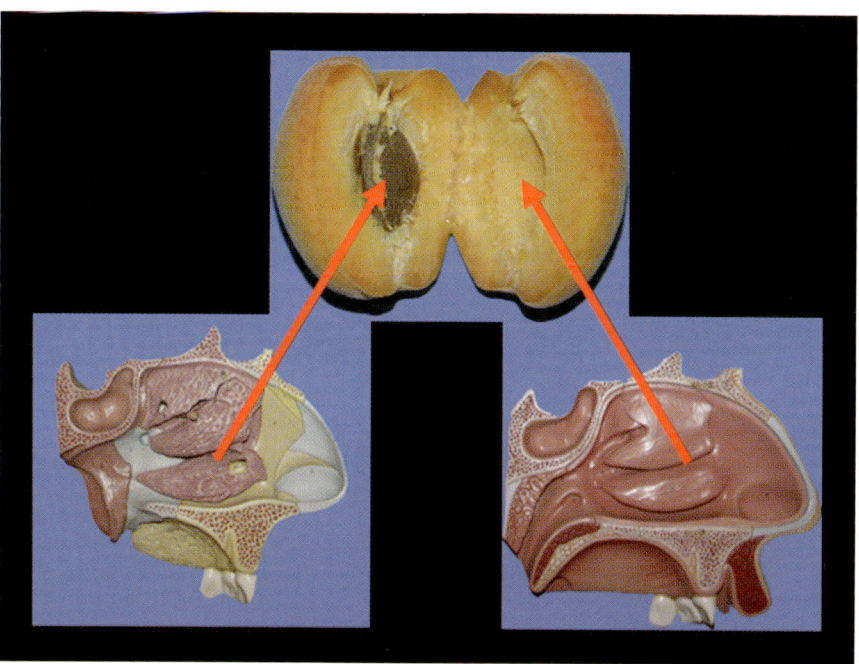

Once the stone is reduced, the pulp and the peel of the fruit should be reduced too. This is the simile with which MIT can be explained to patients during their first visit. We can now proceed to reduce the volume of the two turbinate flaps by using the specific angled scissors.

Reduction and removal of the superior tissue flap of the turbinate.

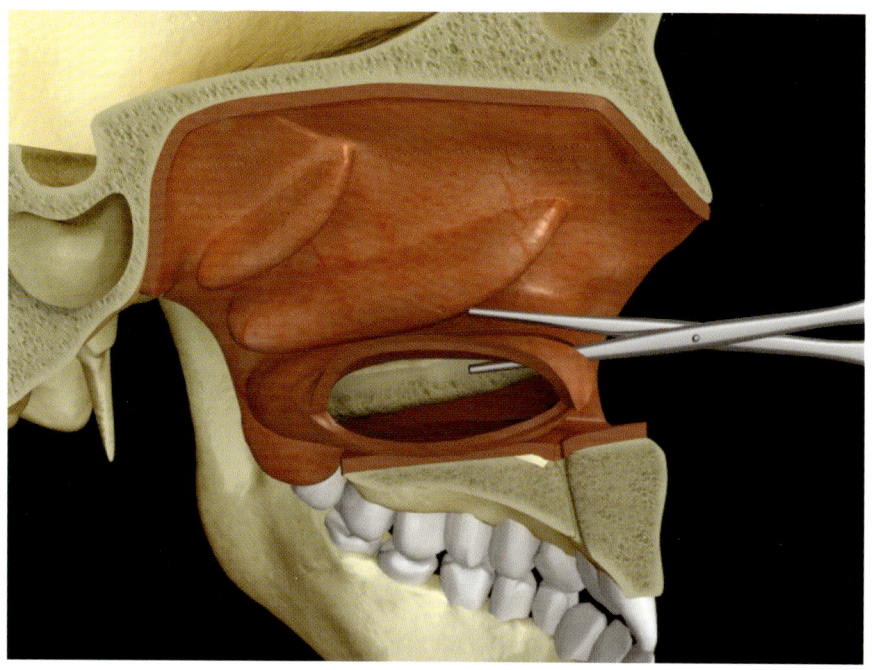

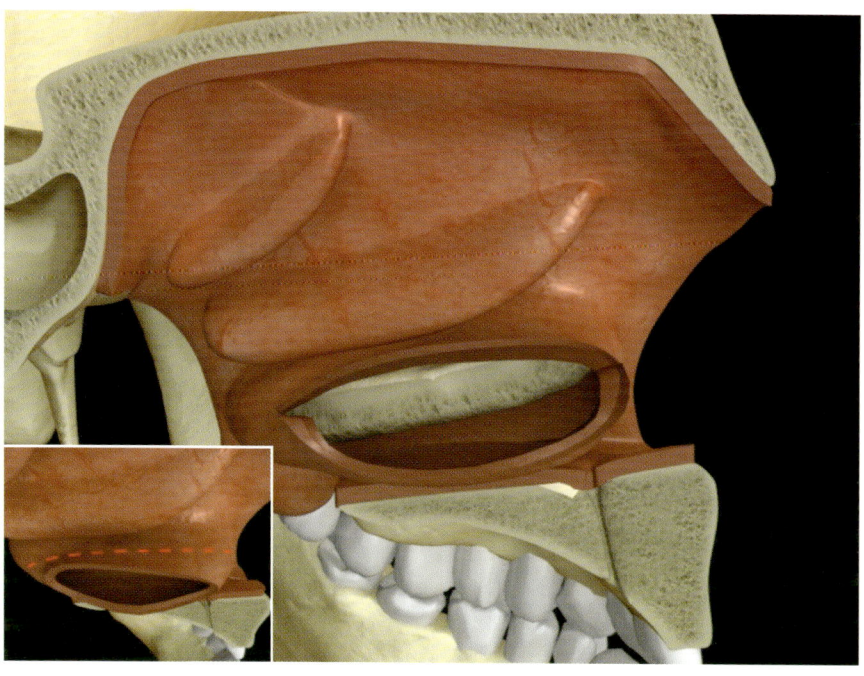

Generally, the thicker part is represented by the lower flap and its removal will obviously turn out to be asymmetric. The removed tissue will have a lozenge shape, looking like a reddish leech.

During this step, by analyzing the removed structures, the tissue changes caused, for instance, by a frequent use of vasoconstrictors may be seen. In this case, a pale and thickened mucosa will be seen, or else the post-treatment degeneration of "hot" techniques may be noticed, as well as the so-called morular degeneration by the irregular edge of the lining mucosa or even by real polypoid degenerations.

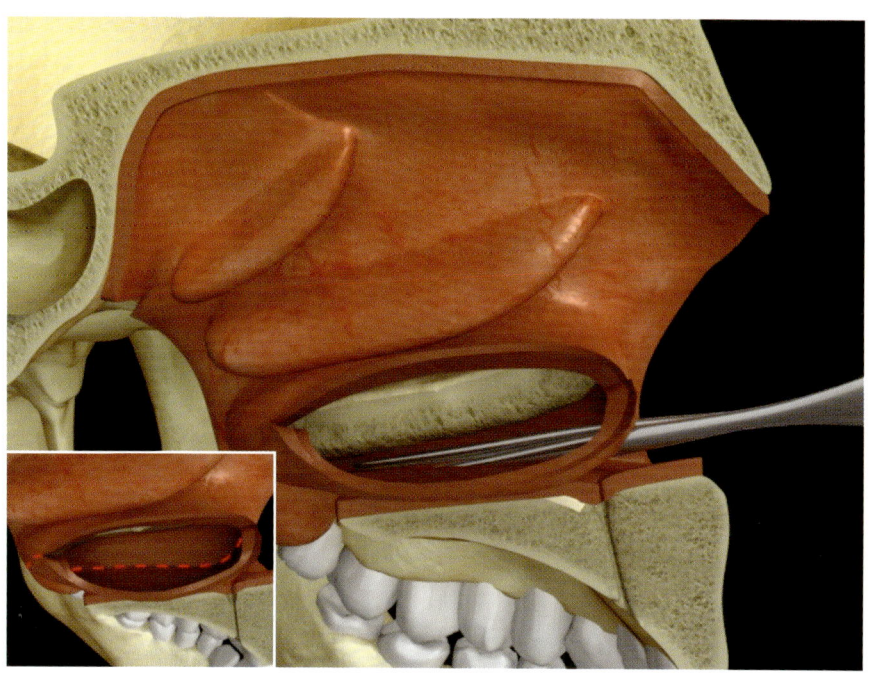

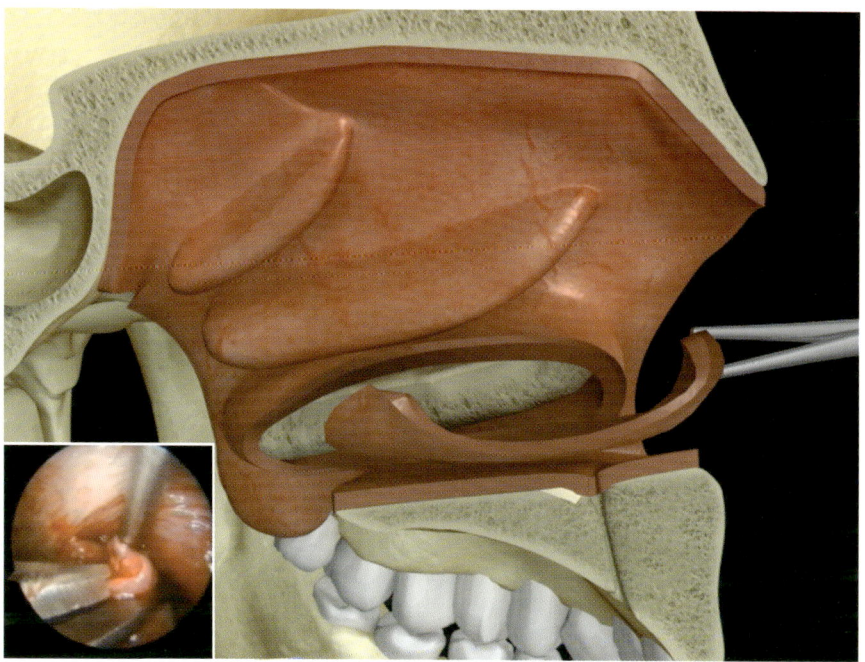

Washings with saline solution are repeatedly performed at each step of rhinoplasty as well as of turbinoplasty procedures.

Before starting the reconstruction of the inferior turbinate with stitches, it is advisable to carry out repeated washing to remove small bone fragments that could lead to complications.

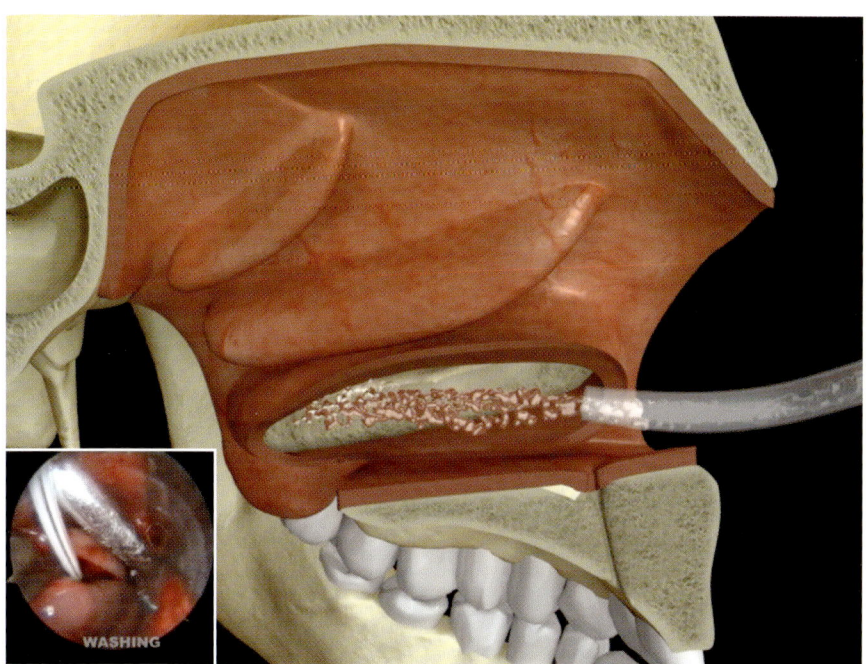

The great advantage of this method, if well executed by suturing the turbinate flaps, is the perfect anatomic restoration, as plastic surgery does in a breast reduction intervention.

This is not only satisfying, but also essential to maintain the breathing air-flow unchanged as much as possible. The suture material used in these cases is an acid polylactic wire with a P3 curved sharp needle. The use of a Castroviejo needle held with thin tapered branches is strongly recommended. When the visibility of the turbinate tail is optimal, a continuous suture may be performed starting from the deep structure and paying attention to joining the flaps as much as possible. Sometimes it is advisable to start the suture with detached stitches, starting from the head of the turbinate. This will simplify the stitching procedure distally at the tail. The upper attachment of the flaps will subsequently allow for a better vision to join the flaps at a deeper level. As a general rule, two wires are used for each turbinate, in order to have a new and sharper needle for the deep suture. The needle may get blunt by crushing against the residual curled bone.

Once turbinate reconstruction is finished, it may be useful to temporarily insert a half n. 8 Merocel buffer until the end of the intervention, whose mild compression will prevent blood storage within the neo-turbinate, facilitating attachment of the flaps to the periosteum. When the septoplasty or sep-torhinoplasty operation is done, the buffers will be removed as they are no longer needed with this method. In the postoperative period, endonasal washings three times daily will guarantee suture absorption in about four weeks.

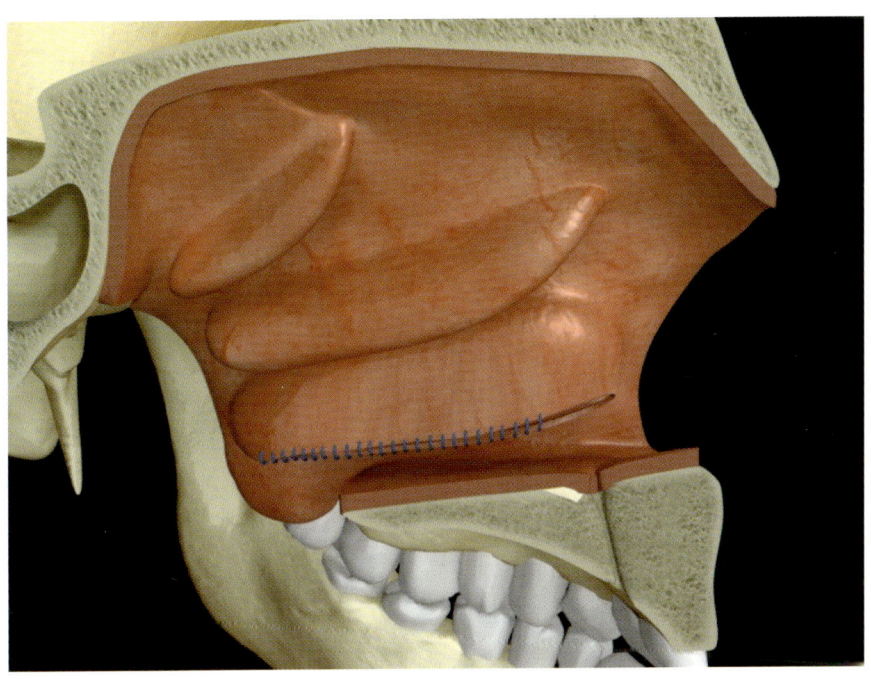

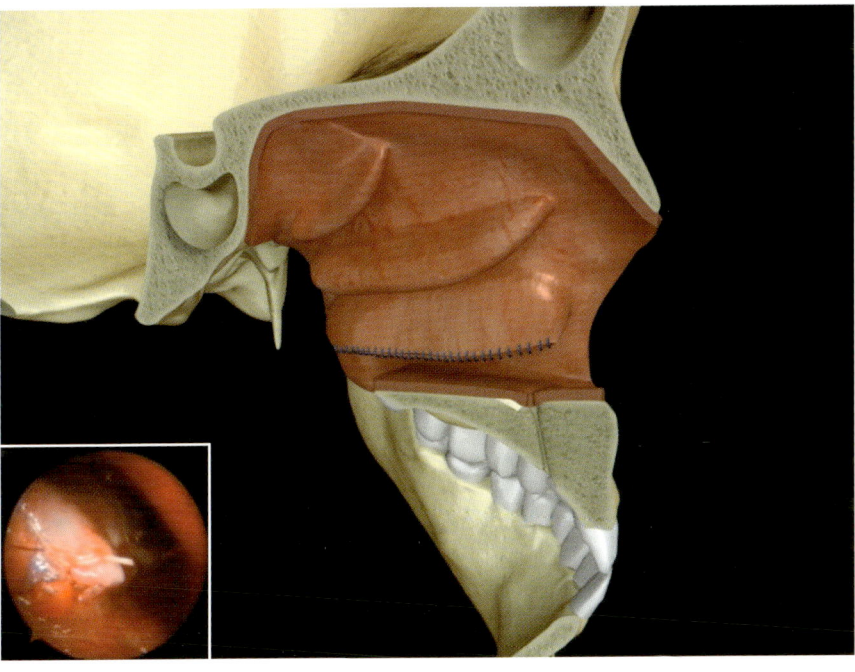

The Concept of "Respiratory Symmetry" **10**

In this chapter the reader will find the essence of nasal surgery interpretation. Inferior turbinate hypertrophy was an unsolved problem before MIT; instead of being the decisive solvers of these health problems, surgeons had to take on more modest and unpretentious tones to explain to the patient the onset of relapse and treatment failure.

Thanks to the logic and common sense that have guided such a new method (i.e. reduction or re-shaping of all three hypertrofied anatomical compartments with tissue reconstruction through a precise suture that avoids buffers and bleeding), MIT has finally solved the essential problem of inferior turbinate hypertrophy. But another, equally important problem remained pending: how to limit any possible extrinsic cause that could favor inferior turbinate hypertrophy. Starting from the assumption that the inferior turbinate always perceives any new uni- or bilateral change in the inspiratory airflow by producing hypertrophy – although with different timings from patient to patient – we must always seek to reproduce "symmetrical" airflows as much as possible.

The reader will now wonder how it may be possible to discuss about "air symmetries" when, from a physiological viewpoint, the result of the so-called "nasal cycle" leads, during daytime, to an obvious asymmetry?

One of the possible interpretations of this phenomenon is to be found in a continuous and alternated automatic control of the functions of these very important organs, the lower turbinates. When several examinations depict a permanent anatomical change, an irreversible hypertrophy process (usually compensatory) has been triggered. The reason for this irreversibility, in spite of denial by some renown surgeons, lies in the fact that hypertrophy starts in the soft tissues, then involves the inferior curled bone (metabolic and bony distraction theory), creating a new anatomic disease that could only be clearly treated through multi-compartmental reductive surgery. MIT is exactly the ideal method for the definitive solution to this disease.

Therefore, experienced rhinoplasty surgeons should always make sure, during the preliminary diagnosis, to check all the anatomical structures that can affect "symmetric" breathing. We have seen how CT scans of the paranasal sinuses can be of great help during this stage; an accurate and targeted assessment of the external nose, by also controlling shape and stability of the nose tip, the convex or concave form of one or both alar or triangular cartilages, as well as any likely diversion or deviation, could become more useful.

In post-traumatic noses (the "boxer's nose" for instance) or in some failed rhinoplasty outcomes, the height and projection of the nasal bridge (saddle nose) as well as the stability or instability of the tip, often totally unsupported with relevant collapse, should be carefully checked.

These alterations in shape create valvular insufficiencies that cannot be ignored. Palpation of tip consistency will reveal the lack of columellar support of the caudal septum, typical of the boxer's nose, but also of many septoplasty outcomes, improperly performed with Cottle's technique.

As far as septal deviations are concerned, CT findings cannot be completely reliable. Radiologists should visit their patients before performing a CT scan. There are, in fact, many caudal septal deviations unrevealed at imaging (because actually, they are caudal cartilages) that could be clearly revealed through an external inspection.

Therefore, asymmetric respiration is mainly caused by the following reasons:
• septal deflection;
• valvular insufficiency;
• stenosing neoformations.

The Control of Relapses in Septal Deviations

11

With regard to the control of septal deviation relapses, an updated system will be illustrated to fix the caudal to the superior maxillary septum and, in particular, to the anterior nasal spine.

It is a particular stitch, which safely and strongly joins together a fragile tissue (the septal cartilage) to another extremely hard and cohesive one (the bone). Furthermore, a second difficulty frequently occurs, caused by the distance between the cartilaginous septum and the bone. This distance (ranging from 1 to 6-7 mm) forms immediately after the removal of the deviated portion at its insertion level in the palatine crest of the superior maxilla. With a regular suture, the difficulty is focused on the ability to tighten the approaching suture properly without tearing the cartilage. Almost always, the assistant must hold the knot using the anatomical clamp before final suture tightening. Gottarelli's "3GK" stitch has solved these problems once and for all.

11.1 Technical Performance

According to personal experience, a 3/0 braided, non-absorbable wire, with a bladed needle (Ethibond, Ethicon) is used. After needle passage through the two sides to be joined, instead of proceeding and knotting the wire, the head of the wire should be passed at least three times around the other end of the wire (dormant). This creates a sort of snaky stitch that has a double purpose: wire locking (keeping it in tension) and creation of a kind of tension-breaker or, better, tension-distributor along the axis of the wire with a "coil", thus preventing cartilage collapse and breakdown, but maintaining its correct position.

The number of turns around the head of the dormant wire should be at least three if the gap between septum and bone is between 0 and 2 mm. For every additional millimeter, an additional turn around the coil should be added; for example, if the distance between the two different tissues is 5 mm, a coil of at least 6 turns should be created.

Of course, once the coil step is completed, the three regular knots of permanent closure will have to be carried out.

With this method there is no possibility to create a relapse for dislocation of septum quadrangular cartilage. With the aim of "balancing" the airflows, any obstacle arising from the ridges and spurs of the osteoseptum will obviously be eliminated. If valvular insufficiency coexists, it will be treated with cartilaginous grafts, such as Sheen spreader grafts, with cartilaginous battens if there is a collapse of the lateral crus or with a transversal graft between the two lateral crura or lateral crural spanning graft (LCSG), as described by Tebbetts.

If polipoyd neoformation or anything else arises, its removal should be carried out, as well as the possibility to perform an enlargement of the meatal ostium, according to the philosophy of Stammberger's functional endoscopic sinus surgery (FESS), should always be strongly taken into consideration.

Conlusions

Several reviews in the literature highlight the success and limitations of the different surgical techniques used in turbinate hypertrophy treatment.

Passali and colleagues have conducted a trial on 457 patients affected by nasal obstruction operated with different techniques, excluding patients with rhinitis and/or infectious sinusitis, nasal septum deviations, polyposis or those who had previously undergone other surgical treatments. At 4 year follow-up on 382 patients, the results of the analysis showed short-term respiratory permeability (in terms of nasal permeability through the assessment of nasal resistance by rhinomanometry and rhinometric volumes detection) when techniques such as electrocautery, cryotherapy and laser therapy were used, that could only be upgraded using turbinectomy.

Another aspect emerging from this study is that the out-patient treatment is worsened by a higher rate of scars and nasal function changes, while submucosal decongestion treatments are often complicated by postoperative bleeding, as well as turbinectomy, even though it stimulates the recovery of mucociliary transport and local production of humoral defense factors. The conclusion of the Italian authors is that the technique of choice in inferior turbinate hypertrophy treatment is the decongestion of the submucosa, better still with lateral dislocation, which is able to restore nasal district activities with the respect of nasal physiology.

Hol et al. reached the same conclusions: turbinoplasty seems to represent the method of choice. Some time later, Willat reintroduced the concept that it must not be identified as the only best technique, but as the right method for all patients with the purpose of obtaining long-term results. This aim has been pursued in the development of the MIT technique, which undoubtedly represents at present the most complete approach for reduction of the inferior turbinate. This technique, associated with structural rhinoplasty and FVTR, has led to a new approach in nose surgery, Global Rhinoplasty (functional and aesthetic), thanks to which a decrease in postoperative bleeding

Paolo Gottarelli, *Modified Inferior Turbinoplasty* © Springer-Verlag Italia 2012

risk may be attained by completely eliminating the use of the so-dreaded swabs and by improving the quality of patient's life after surgery. A method capable, after all, of combining clinical needs with the patient's aesthetic expectations, with compliance levels never obtained before.

Suggested Reading

Balbach L, Trinkel V, Guldner C, Bien S, Teymoortash A, Werner JA, Bremke M (2011) Radiological examinations of the anatomy of the inferior turbinate using digital volume tomography (DVT). Rhinology 49:248-252

Batra PS, Seiden AM, Smith TL (2009) Surgical management of adult inferior turbinate hypertrophy: a systematic review of the evidence. Laryngoscope 119:1819-1827

Bhandarkar ND, Smith TL (2010) Outcomes of surgery for inferior turbinate hypertrophy. Curr Opin Otolaryngol Head Neck Surg 18:49-53

Caffier PP, Frieler K, Scherer H, Sedlmaier B, Göktas O (2008) Rhinitis medicamentosa: therapeutic effect of diode laser inferior turbinate reduction on nasal obstruction and decongestant abuse. Am J Rhinol 22:433-439

Cavaliere M, Mottola G, Iemma M (2005) Comparison of the effectiveness and safety of radiofrequency turbinoplasty and traditional surgical technique in treatment of inferior turbinate hypertrophy. Otolaryngol Head Neck Surg 133:972-978

Chen XB, Lee HP, Chong VF, Wang de Y (2010) Numerical simulation of the effects of inferior turbinate surgery on nasal airway heating capacity. Am J Rhinol Allergy 24:118-122

Chusakul S, Choktaweekarn T, Snidvongs K, Phannaso C, Aeumjaturapat S (2011) Effect of the KTP laser in inferior turbinate surgery on eosinophil influx in allergic rhinitis. Otolaryngol Head Neck Surg 144:237-240

Feldman EM, Koshy JC, Chike-Obi CJ, Hatef DA, Bullocks JM, Stal S (2010) Contemporary techniques in inferior turbinate reduction: survey results of the American Society for Aesthetic Plastic Surgery. Aesthet Surg J 30:672-679

Glorig A, Wheeler DE, House HP (1958) Your ear and nose. AMA Arch Ind Health 17:81-85

Greywoode JD, Van Abel K, Pribitkin EA (2010) Ultrasonic bone aspirator turbinoplasty: a novel approach for management of inferior turbinate hypertrophy. Laryngoscope 120 Suppl 4:239

Gottarelli P, Righini S (1996) 8-year experience with force vector rhinoplasty by J.B. Tebbetts: comparative results. Acta Otorhinolaryngol Ital 16:248-253

Gupta V, Singh H, Gupta M, Singh S (2011) Dislocation of the inferior turbinates: a rare complication of nasal surgery, presenting as obstructive sleep apnea. J Laryngol Otol 125:859-860

Hol MK, Huizing EH (2000) Treatment of inferior turbinate pathology: a review and critical evaluation of the different techniques. Rhinology 38:157-166

House HP (1951) Submucous resection of the interior turbinal bone. Laryngoscope 61:637-648

Jose J, Coatesworth AP (2010) Inferior turbinate surgery for nasal obstruction in allergic rhinitis after failed medical treatment. Cochrane Database Syst Rev. 12:CD005235

Lee DH, Kim EH (2010) Microdebrider-assisted versus laser-assisted turbinate reduction: comparison of improvement in nasal airway according to type of turbinate hypertrophy. Ear Nose Throat J. 89:541-545

Lee HP, Garlapati RR, Chong VF, Wang DY (2011) Comparison between effects of various partial inferior turbinectomy options on nasal airflow: a computer simulation study. Comput Methods Biomech Biomed Engin Sept 14 (in corso di pubblicazione)

Lilja M, Virkkula P (2010) [Surgical techniques of the inferior nasal turbinates in the treatment of nasal obstruction]. Duodecim 126:2023-2031

Mabry RL (1988) Inferior turbinoplasty: patient selection, technique, and long-term consequences. Otolaryngol Head Neck Surg 98:60-66

Meneghini F, Gottarelli P (2002) Lateral crus sculpturing in open rhinoplasty: the Delicate Alar Clamp. Aesthetic Plast Surg 26:73-77

Nurse LA, Duncavage JA (2009) Surgery of the inferior and middle turbinates. Otolaryngol Clin North Am 42:295-309

Passali D, Lauriello M, De Filippi A, Bellussi L (1995) Comparative study of most recent surgical techniques for the treatment of the hypertrophy of inferior turbinates. Acta Otorhinolaryngol Ital 15:219-228

Passali D, Passali FM, Damiani V, Passali GC, Bellussi L (2003) Treatment of inferior turbinate hypertrophy: a randomized clinical trial. Ann Otol Rhinol Laryngol 112:683-688

Pittore B, Al Safi W, Jarvis SJ (2011) Concha bullosa of the inferior turbinate: an unusual cause of nasal obstruction. Acta Otorhinolaryngol Ital 31:47-49

Pollock RA, Rohrich RJ. Inferior turbinate surgery: an adjunct to successful treatment of nasal obstruction in 408 patients (1984) Plast Reconstr Surg 74:227-236

Tebbetts JB (1998) Primary rhinoplasty: a new approach to logic and techniques. Mosby, St Louis

Toriumi DM (1993) Open structure rhinoplasty. Facial Plast Surg Clin North Am 1:1

Warwick-Brown NP, Marks NJ (1987) Turbinate surgery: how effective is it? A longterm assessment. ORL J Otorhinolaryngol Relat Spec 49:314-320

Willat D (2009) The evidence for reducing inferior turbinates. Rhinology 47:237-246

About the Author

Academic Activities

Born in Bologna in 1952, Paolo Gottarelli graduated in 1978 in Medicine and Surgery with honors in the same city. Later on, he specialized in plastic surgery and dentistry.
From 1980 to 1996 he was hospital assistant and primary aid at the Division of Plastic Surgery at the Rizzoli Orthopedic Institute in Bologna.
Subsequently, he obtained further post-graduate diplomas in biomaterials, cosmetic surgery and nasal surgery.
From 1992 to 2007 he worked with a fixed-term contract as Professor of Aesthetic and Functional Corrective Surgical Techniques of the nasal pyramid at the University of Ferrara Department of Otolaryngology directed by Charles Calearo.
From 1992 to 1995 he worked with a fixed-term contract as Professor of Plastic Surgery principles at the School of Specialization in Physical Medicine and Rehabilitation – University of Bologna.
From 1992 to 1994 he worked with a fixed-term contract as Professor of Surgery of oral pre-cancer at the School of Dentistry and specialization in Dental Prosthesis at the University of Bologna.
From 1992 to 1993 he worked with a fixed-term contract as Professor at the Higher Institute of Holistic Medicine and Ecology at the University of Urbino.

Professional Activities

In 1989, he introduced for the first time in Italy the innovative Septorhinoplasty technique by John B. Tebbetts, Dallas.
Since 1991 he was interested in Plastic Surgery computer application, with particular respect for the informed consent.
From 1992 to 2008, in addition to the ordinary academic activities, he held CME accredited lectures on Septorhinoplasty, Outpatient Surgery and Lip Surgery.
In 1994 he won the 1st prize for best performance at the National Congress of Videoplasty Surgery of the Italian Hospital Surgeons Association (ACOI, *Associazione Chirurghi Opedalieri Italiani*) with a multimedia video about Tebbetts' Rhinoplasty technique.
In 1996, at the 45th National Congress of Plastic Surgery, he organized the "Plastic surgeon and computer" workshop.

In 1997, he was the Chairman of debates about the peculiarities of patients who undergo plastic surgery at the Informatics Fair "Future Show 2997". In June, he ran the first multimedia video lecture on Open Septorhinoplasty according to Tebbetts' method.

In 1997 he developed the modified inferior turbinoplasty (MIT), an innovative method of reshaping the inferior turbinates with 4,000 case reports.

In 1998 he was invited to hold a magisterial lesson about Force Vector Tip Rhinoplasty (FVTR) at the 13th training course of Cosmetic Surgery (monothematic course of Primary and Secondary Rhinoplasty) in Trieste.

In 2002 he was invited for two lectures at the International Conference of Rhinoplasty, Dubrovnik.

In 2003 he participated in the 5th Symposium on Aesthetic Plastic Surgery in Barcelona, where he performed some Rhinoplasty surgeries at the Teknon Medical Center. In this occasion he showed for the first time his MIT technique.

In 2004 he attended the 14th International Course on Plastic and Aesthetic Surgery, Barcelona, chaired by Jaime Planas, where he presented four reports on nasal correction techniques he developed and performed some live interventions at the Clinica Planas.

In 2005 he participated in the 23rd International Annual Symposium of Plastic Surgery-Aesthetics of Guadalajara in Mexico, chaired by José Guerrero Santos, where he illustrated his innovative method on Global Rhinoplasty and modified inferior turbinoplasty.

To date, he is Director and Lecturer of numerous workshops in different Plastic Surgery fields. In 2010 he also had a video made about MIT. The number of patients operated with this technique has nowadays reached 5,000.

Printed in December 2011